Achilles Tendon Pathology

Editor

PAUL DAYTON

CLINICS IN PODIATRIC MEDICINE AND SURGERY

www.podiatric.theclinics.com

Consulting Editor
THOMAS ZGONIS

April 2017 • Volume 34 • Number 2

ELSEVIER

1600 John F. Kennedy Boulevard • Suite 1800 • Philadelphia, Pennsylvania, 19103-2899

http://www.theclinics.com

CLINICS IN PODIATRIC MEDICINE AND SURGERY Volume 34, Number 2
April 2017 ISSN 0891-8422, ISBN-13: 978-0-323-52429-2

Editor: Lauren Boyle
Developmental Editor: Alison Swety

Clinics in Podiatric Medicine and Surgery (ISSN 0891-8422) is published quarterly by Elsevier Inc., 360 Park Avenue South, New York, NY 10010-1710. Months of issue are January, April, July, and October. Business and Editorial Offices: 1600 John F. Kennedy Blvd., Ste. 1800, Philadelphia, PA 19103-2899. Customer Service Office: 3251 Riverport Lane, Maryland Heights, MO 63043. Periodicals postage paid at New York, NY and additional mailing offices. Subscription prices are $288.00 per year for US individuals, $518.00 per year for US institutions, $100.00 per year for US students and residents, $374.00 per year for Canadian individuals, $626.00 for Canadian institutions, $439.00 for international individuals, $626.00 per year for international institutions and $220.00 per year for Canadian and foreign students/residents. To receive student/resident rate, orders must be accompanied by name of affiliated institution, date of term, and the *signature* of program/residency coordinator on institution letterhead. Orders will be billed at individual rate until proof of status is received. Foreign air speed delivery is included in all *Clinics* subscription prices. All prices are subject to change without notice. POSTMASTER: Send address changes to *Clinics in Podiatric Medicine and Surgery*, Elsevier Health Sciences Division, Subscription Customer Service, 3251 Riverport Lane, Maryland Heights, MO 63043. **Customer Service: 1-800-654-2452 (US). From outside of the US, call 314-447-8871. Fax: 314-447-8029. E-mail: JournalsCustomerService-usa@elsevier.com (for print support); JournalsOnlineSupport-usa@elsevier. com (for online support).**

Reprints. For copies of 100 or more of articles in this publication, please contact the Commercial Reprints Department, Elsevier Inc., 360 Park Avenue South, New York, NY 10010-1710. Tel.: 212-633-3874; Fax: 212-633-3820; E-mail: reprints@elsevier.com.

Clinics in Podiatric Medicine and Surgery is covered in *MEDLINE/PubMed (Index Medicus)* and *EMBASE/Excerpta Medica.*

CLINICS IN PODIATRIC MEDICINE AND SURGERY

CONSULTING EDITOR
THOMAS ZGONIS, DPM, FACFAS

Contributors

CONSULTING EDITOR

THOMAS ZGONIS, DPM, FACFAS
Professor and Director, Externship and Reconstructive Foot and Ankle Fellowship
Programs, Division of Podiatric Medicine and Surgery, Department of Orthopaedics,
University of Texas Health Science Center San Antonio, San Antonio, Texas

EDITOR

PAUL DAYTON, DPM, MS, FACFAS
UnityPoint Clinic Foot and Ankle, Assistant Professor, College of Podiatric Medicine and
Surgery, Des Moines University, Fort Dodge, Iowa

AUTHORS

MARK J. BULLOCK, DPM, AACFAS
Foot and Ankle Surgeon, Saginaw Valley Bone and Joint Center, Saginaw, Michigan

BRADLY W. BUSSEWITZ, DPM, FACFAS
Steindler Orthopedic Clinic, Iowa City, Iowa

GAGE M. CAUDELL, DPM, FACFAS
Fort Wayne Orthopedics, Fort Wayne, Indiana

DEREK CLEWLEY, DPT, OCS, FAAOMPT
Assistant Professor, Division of Doctor of Physical Therapy, Duke University, Durham,
North California

JAMES DAVIES, MD
Orthopedic Surgeon, Department of Orthopedics, University of South Carolina, Columbia,
South Carolina

PAUL DAYTON, DPM, MS, FACFAS
UnityPoint Clinic Foot and Ankle, Assistant Professor, College of Podiatric Medicine and
Surgery, Des Moines University, Fort Dodge, Iowa

WILLIAM T. DeCARBO, DPM, FACFAS
Foot and Ankle Surgeon, The Orthopedic Group, Belle Vernon, Pennsylvania

PATRICK A. DeHEER, DPM
Staff, Surgery Department, Indiana University Health North Hospital, Carmel, Indiana;
Staff, Surgery Department, Johnson Memorial Hospital, Franklin, Indiana; Clinical
Instructor (Adjunct Track), Department of Podiatric Medicine and Radiology, Rosalind
Franklin University of Medicine and Science, North Chicago, Illinois

JASON GEORGE DeVRIES, DPM, FACFAS
Foot and Ankle Surgeon, Orthopedics & Sports Medicine, BayCare Clinic, Green Bay, Wisconsin

MINDI FEILMEIER, DPM, FACFAS
Assistant Professor, College of Podiatric Medicine and Surgery, Des Moines University, Des Moines, Iowa

ANDREW J. FRIEDMANN, MD
Chief Resident PGY-4, Department of Orthopaedics, Robert C. Byrd Health Sciences Center, West Virginia University, Morgantown, West Virginia

ANDREW E. HANSELMAN, MD
Chief Resident PGY-4, Department of Orthopaedics, Robert C. Byrd Health Sciences Center, West Virginia University, Morgantown, West Virginia

MERRELL KAUWE, DPM
Foot and Ankle Department, UnityPoint Trinity Regional Medical Center, Fort Dodge, Iowa

LACE LUEDKE, DPT, PhD, OCS, CSCS
Lecturer, Kinesiology Department, University of Wisconsin-Oshkosh, Oshkosh, Wisconsin

JAMES M. MAHONEY, DPM
Professor of Podiatric Medicine, College of Podiatric Medicine and Surgery, Des Moines University, Des Moines, Iowa

SHANE McCLINTON, DPT, OCS, FAAOMPT, CSCS
Assistant Professor, Doctor of Physical Therapy Program, Des Moines University, Des Moines, Iowa

WILL MELTON, MD
Orthopedic Surgeon, Department of Orthopedics, University of South Carolina, Columbia, South Carolina

CRYSTAL L. RAMANUJAM, DPM, MSc
Assistant Professor/Clinical, Division of Podiatric Medicine and Surgery, Department of Orthopaedics, University of Texas Health Science Center San Antonio, San Antonio, Texas

ROBERT D. SANTROCK, MD
Assistant Professor, Chief of Foot and Ankle Orthopaedics, Department of Orthopaedics, Robert C. Byrd Health Sciences Center, West Virginia University, Morgantown, West Virginia

BRANDON M. SCHARER, DPM, FACFAS
Foot and Ankle Surgeon, Orthopedics & Sports Medicine, BayCare Clinic, Green Bay, Wisconsin

WILLIAM BRET SMITH, DO, MSc, FAOAO
Director of Foot and Ankle Division, Assistant Professor, Department of Orthopedics, University of South Carolina, Columbia, South Carolina

BENJAMIN J. SUMMERHAYS, DPM, FACFAS
Clinical Assistant Professor, Orthopaedic Surgery, University of Missouri Health, Columbia, Missouri

THOMAS ZGONIS, DPM, FACFAS
Professor and Director, Externship and Reconstructive Foot and Ankle Fellowship Programs, Division of Podiatric Medicine and Surgery, Department of Orthopaedics, University of Texas Health Science Center San Antonio, San Antonio, Texas

Contents

Preface: The Essential Achilles   xv

Paul Dayton

Anatomic, Vascular, and Mechanical Overview of the Achilles Tendon   107

Paul Dayton

The Achilles tendon is the strongest and thickest tendon in the body and is subjected to unique forces during the activities of living. A variety of pathologic processes have been identified causing clinical symptoms in patients of all ages. A detailed understanding of Achilles anatomy is necessary to understand the pathologic process that are seen in the tendon. As with all medical topics and conditions, our understanding is evolving as new research sheds light on pathologic processes involved with the Achilles tendon. This article reviews the anatomic, histologic, hemodynamic, and mechanical properties of the Achilles tendon and associated muscle structures.

Imaging Techniques and Indications   115

James M. Mahoney

 Video content accompanies this article at http://www.podiatric.theclinics.com.

This article evaluates the utility of radiography, ultrasonography, and MRI in diagnosing Achilles tendon injuries. It reviews the pertinent anatomy of the Achilles and associated structures, and signs of disorder with each imaging technique. The economics of use ultrasonography and MRI are discussed. They should serve as complementary diagnostic tools, with ultrasonography the first choice because of its ease of use, ability to view dynamic function, and cost. However, clinical examination is often best for diagnosis; MRI and ultrasonography often should be considered only when the diagnosis is confounding or a patient does not respond to recommended conservative care.

Noninsertional Achilles Tendinopathy Pathologic Background and Clinical Examination   129

Mindi Feilmeier

The term tendinopathy includes a series of pathologies, all of which have a combination of pain, swelling, and impaired performance. The terms tendinosis, tendinitis and peritendinitis are all within the main heading of tendinopathy; this terminology provides a more accurate understanding of the condition and highlights the uniformity of clinical findings while distinguishing the individual histopathological findings of each condition. Understanding the clinical features and the underlying histopathology leads to a more accurate clinical diagnosis and subsequent treatment selection. Misuse of the term tendinitis can lead to the underestimation of chronic degenerative nature of many tendinopathies, affecting the treatment selection.

Nonsurgical Management of Midsubstance Achilles Tendinopathy   137

Shane McClinton, Lace Luedke, and Derek Clewley

Midsubstance Achilles tendinopathy is one of the most common lower leg conditions. Most patients can recover with nonsurgical treatment that focuses on tendon loading exercises and, when necessary, symptom modulating treatments such as topical, oral, or injected medication, ice, shoe inserts, manual therapy, stretching, taping, or low-level laser. If unresponsive to initial management, a small percentage of patients may consider shockwave or sclerosing treatment and possibly surgery.

Midsubstance Tendinopathy, Percutaneous Techniques (Platelet-Rich Plasma, Extracorporeal Shock Wave Therapy, Prolotherapy, Radiofrequency Ablation)   161

William Bret Smith, Will Melton, and James Davies

The focus of this article is to present the current options available for noninvasive and percutaneous treatment options for noninsertional Achilles tendinopathy. An attempt is made to offer recommendations for both the treatment techniques as well as postprocedure protocols to be considered. Additionally, because there are numerous treatment options in this category, the different techniques are summarized in a chart format with a short list of pros and cons as well as the levels of evidence in the literature to support the different modalities.

Midsubstance Tendinopathy, Surgical Management   175

William T. DeCarbo and Mark J. Bullock

Noninsertional Achilles tendinopathy often responds to nonoperative treatment. When nonoperative treatment fails, the clinician must distinguish between paratendinopathy and noninsertional tendinopathy. In paratendinopathy, myofibroblasts synthesize collagen, causing adhesions, and the paratenon may be released or excised. If a core area of tendinopathy is identified on MRI, the area is excised longitudinally and repaired with a side-to-side suture. If greater than 50% of the tendon diameter is excised, the authors recommend a short flexor hallucis longus tendon transfer with an interference screw. A turndown flap of the gastrocnemius aponeurosis is also described with good results.

Insertional Achilles Tendinopathy   195

Gage M. Caudell

Posterior heel pain is a common condition of the foot and ankle and is seen in a variety of foot types. Nonoperative treatment methods consisting of shoes inserts, heel lifts, stretching, physical therapy, nonsteroidal antiinflammatory drugs, eccentric strength training, and other modalities have been shown to have mixed results. When indicated, surgical repair can produce good long-term results. Complications, although uncommon, most commonly result from wound healing complications.

Equinus and Lengthening Techniques   207

Patrick A. DeHeer

Equinus is linked to most lower extremity biomechanically related disorders. Defining equinus as ankle joint dorsiflexion less than 5° of dorsiflexion with the knee extended is the basis for evaluation and management of the deformity. Consistent evaluation methodology using a goniometer with the subtalar joint in neutral position and midtarsal joint supinated while dorsiflexing the ankle with knee extended provides a consistent clinical examination. For equinus deformity with an associated disorder, comprehensive treatment mandates treatment of the equinus deformity. Surgical treatment of equinus offers multiple procedures but the Baumann gastrocnemius recession is preferred based on deformity correction without weakness.

Acute Achilles Tendon Rupture: Clinical Evaluation, Conservative Management, and Early Active Rehabilitation   229

Merrell Kauwe

The Achilles tendon (AT) is the strongest, largest, and most commonly ruptured tendon in the human body. Physical examination provides high sensitivity and specificity. Imaging studies are not recommended unless there are equivocal findings in the physical examination. Recent studies have shown that the risk of re-rupture is negated with implementation of functional rehabilitation protocols. Heterogeneity in study design makes conclusions on the specifics of functional rehabilitation protocols difficult; however, it is clear that early weight bearing and early controlled mobilization lead to better patient outcome and satisfaction in both surgically and conservatively treated populations.

Acute Rupture Open Repair Techniques   245

Robert D. Santrock, Andrew J. Friedmann, and Andrew E. Hanselman

Achilles tendon injuries can be serious injuries requiring either operative or nonoperative management. For appropriate surgical candidates, operative intervention may provide lower rerupture rates and adequate end-to-end tendon healing. Our preference is an open Achilles tendon repair, specifically a limited open technique using the PARS device (Arthrex, Naples, FL). Postoperatively, we use functional rehabilitation and early range of motion. Although the current literature remains controversial regarding operative versus nonoperative management, the authors have obtained satisfactory results in appropriately chosen surgical candidates.

Acute Achilles Rupture Percutaneous Repair: Approach, Materials, Techniques   251

Jason George DeVries, Brandon M. Scharer, and Benjamin J. Summerhays

Closed traumatic Achilles tendon rupture is a common injury, especially in the aging athlete. Traditionally open repair has been recognized to offer a lower rerupture rate compared with nonoperative methods but with a higher complication rate. Percutaneous repair has been described to offer the benefits of open repair while avoiding the complications. The sural nerve is potentially susceptible to injury, and specialized instrumentation has been developed to avoid this event. This article discusses several techniques of minimally invasive Achilles tendon repair. Many authors have evaluated these techniques and the results are discussed here.

Repair of Neglected Achilles Rupture   263

Bradly W. Bussewitz

Acute Achilles tendon ruptures is routinely missed or undertreated, leading to functional deficits. The neglected Achilles ruptures often requires surgical repair to regain functional improvement. The tendon retraction and resultant necessary debridement of the rupture site leads to difficulty completing end-to-end repair. Advanced techniques, including fascial advancements, tendon transfers, and use of allografts, allow the treating surgeon many viable repair options for the neglected Achilles presentation. The article describes the neglected Achilles tendon, including the nature of the problem, repair options, surgical technique, and a discussion of the surgical outcomes.

**Surgical Correction of the Achilles Tendon for Diabetic Foot Ulcerations and
Charcot Neuroarthropathy**   275

Crystal L. Ramanujam and Thomas Zgonis

Achilles tendon pathologic conditions are implicated in contributing to the development of many diabetic foot complications including diabetic foot ulceration and Charcot neuroarthropathy. Surgical correction of the diabetic equinus deformity has been studied as an isolated or adjunctive treatment when dealing with difficult-to-close diabetic foot ulcerations or when surgically addressing the diabetic Charcot neuroarthropathy foot or ankle. This article reviews the most common indications, complications, and surgical procedures for equinus correction by either a tendo-Achilles lengthening or gastrocnemius recession for the management of diabetic foot conditions.

Index   281

CLINICS IN PODIATRIC MEDICINE AND SURGERY

FORTHCOMING ISSUES

July 2017
Foot and Ankle Arthrodesis
John J. Stapleton, *Editor*

October 2017
Surgical Advances in Ankle Arthritis
Alan Ng, *Editor*

January 2018
**New Technologies in Foot and Ankle
Surgery**
Stephen A. Brigido, *Editor*

RECENT ISSUES

January 2017
**The Diabetic Charcot Foot and Ankle:
A Multidisciplinary Team Approach**
Thomas Zgonis, *Editor*

October 2016
**Current Update on Foot and Ankle
Arthroscopy**
Sean T. Grambart, *Editor*

July 2016
**Dermatological Manifestations of the
Lower Extremity**
Tracey C. Vlahovic, *Editor*

RELATED INTEREST

Foot and Ankle Clinics, March 2014 (Vol. 19, Issue 1)
Tendon Transfers and Treatment Strategies in Foot and Ankle Surgery
Bruce E. Cohen, *Editor*
Available at: http://www.foot.theclinics.com/

Preface

The Essential Achilles

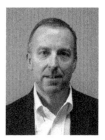

Paul Dayton, DPM, MS, FACFAS
Editor

The Achilles tendon is the largest tendon in the body and is expected to endure biomechanical forces beyond almost any other biological soft tissue structure. The Achilles is essential for normal ambulation and performs both a stabilizing and a propulsive function without which many basic activities of daily living are impossible. As noted in the famous fable of the tendon's name, loss of the function of this vital tendon can have disastrous effects on human function. From acute trauma to degenerative tendinosis, the Achilles tendon is affected by a diverse group of processes. As our understanding of tissue biology, response to injury, and response to therapy expands, we are able to better serve the needs of our patients with Achilles tendon afflictions. New and novel therapies are changing our outlook on injuries and degenerative conditions once thought to be incurable and are offering hope to providers and patients for faster and more complete recovery. One dramatic change I have seen during my 30-year tour in the medical profession is the importance of activity during recovery to direct and improve tissue healing. Gone are the prolonged periods of immobilization that we thought were protecting patients from harm during recovery, and in place, we have a new understanding of the benefits of early and active recovery, which results in quicker and more complete recovery of the tissues and the patient. It has been my pleasure to act as guest editor for this issue of *Clinics in Podiatric Medicine and Surgery*. I would like to offer a heartfelt thank-you to each of the section authors,

Clin Podiatr Med Surg 34 (2017) xv–xvi
http://dx.doi.org/10.1016/j.cpm.2017.01.001
0891-8422/17/© 2017 Published by Elsevier Inc.

who gave their time to present interesting and clinically useful information for all of us to better serve our patients' needs.

Paul Dayton, DPM, MS, FACFAS
UnityPoint Clinic Foot and Ankle
College of Podiatric Medicine
and Surgery
Des Moines University
804 Kenyon Road, Suite 310
Fort Dodge, IA 50501, USA

E-mail address:
daytonp@me.com

Anatomic, Vascular, and Mechanical Overview of the Achilles Tendon

Paul Dayton, DPM, MS

KEYWORDS

• Achilles • Anatomy • Tendon • Biomechanics

KEY POINTS

- The anatomic and histologic properties of the Achilles tendon are directly related to resistance to mechanical damage and subsequent pathologic processes as well as tendon healing.
- Gastrocnemius and soleus anatomy have a direct effect on many pathologic processes in the foot and ankle.
- Experimental data indicating uniform hemodynamic flow throughout the Achilles tendon has challenged the widespread notion that ischemia is a primary etiology of pathology and rupture in the central portion of the tendon, which is based on a circumstantial association with an anatomic watershed.

GROSS ANATOMY

The Achilles is composed of the conjoined tendons of the gastrocnemius, soleus, and occasionally plantaris muscles.[1,2] These associated muscles and the Achilles tendon make up the superficial posterior compartment of the leg. The gastrocnemius muscle is the most superficial component of the triceps surae. The medial and lateral heads of the gastrocnemius arise from the femoral condyles. The medial head originates from behind the medial supracondylar line and adductor tubercle, superior to the medial femoral condyle. The lateral head originates from the posterior aspect of the lateral femoral condyle superior and posterior to the lateral epicondyle, as well as from a portion of the lateral lip of the linea aspera superior to the lateral condyle. The medial head is larger, longer, and extends farther distally than the lateral head. Both heads share an additional origin from the posterior aspect of the knee capsule termed the popliteal ligament. The deep surface of the muscle is tendinous and intimately approximated to the soleus muscle. Deep to both heads may lie bursae. The gastrocnemius

Financial Disclosure: The authors have nothing to disclose.
UnityPoint Clinic Foot and Ankle, College of Podiatric Medicine and Surgery, Des Moines University, 804 Kenyon Road Suite 310, Fort Dodge, IA 50501, USA
E-mail address: daytonp@me.com

heads are large, fusiform bodies that join in the midcalf to form a wide aponeurosis at the muscle's distal aspect. The heads form a tendinous raphe where they meet midline and communicate with the deep, anterior aspect of the aponeurosis. This aponeurosis continues distally as a component of the Achilles tendon.

The soleus muscle is a broad, flat, pennate muscle that arises entirely from below the knee. The muscle lies deep to the gastrocnemius muscle within the superficial posterior compartment of the leg and is housed between 2 aponeurotic lamellae with the posterior aponeurosis beginning more proximally than that of the gastrocnemius. Muscle origins include the head and proximal fourth of the posterior fibula, the oblique line and middle third of the medial tibial border, and the fibrous arch between the 2. The gross muscle is wider and extends more distally than the gastrocnemius with fibers joining centrally in a posterior aponeurosis or intramuscular tendon, which promotes a bipennate arrangement of muscle fibers. This central intramuscular tendon merges distally to form a component of the Achilles tendon. Between gastrocnemius and soleus muscles lies a layer of dense fibrous connective tissue with a film of loose connective tissue between the each of the layers. The posterior aponeurosis of the soleus is the largest contributory component of the Achilles tendon.

The plantaris muscle is variable in size and absent in 6% to 8% of individuals.[2] The plantaris originates from the superior aspect of the lateral femoral condyle. The muscle belly runs medially and continues as a long tendon that extends distally between the gastrocnemius and soleus to insert on the medial border of the Achilles tendon.

The nerve supply to the gastrocsoleus is derived from tibial branches proximally. The Achilles tendon has sparse innervation from several sources arising from the paratendinous soft tissues. The sural nerve is a main contributor to tendon and peritendon structures and is at risk for injury during surgical procedures because of its proximity to the tendon and aponeurosis posteriorly.

The Achilles tendon begins at the musculotendinous junction of the gastrocnemius and soleus muscles with typical full incorporation occurring approximately 8 to 10 cm above the calcaneal insertion site.[1] In total, the Achilles tendon is approximately 15 cm in length and begins flattened at the musculotendinous junction and becomes rounded approximately 4 cm from the calcaneus. The anterior and medial aspects of the tendon receive fibers from the soleus, and the posterior aspect is derived from gastrocnemius fibers. The contributions and proportions from both the gastrocnemius and soleus are variable. As fibers travel distally, they rotate 90° such that gastrocnemius fibers attach laterally and posteriorly, whereas the fibers of the soleus attach medially and anteriorly. This spiraling has been shown to result in less fiber buckling when the tendon is lax and less deformation when tension is applied to the tendon.[3] At its insertion site, the tendon flattens and broadens into a deltoid-type of attachment and develops an anterior concavity before inserting along the middle third of the posterior aspect of the calcaneus. The surface of the distal tendon that overlies the calcaneus is composed of fibrocartilage. Underneath the tendon lies the retrocalcaneal bursa, which is interpositioned between the tendon and the posterior calcaneal tuberosity. At the distal-most insertion of the tendon, some collagen fibers form Sharpey fibers and become continuous with fibrous tissue overlying the calcaneus.

There is no true synovial sheath surrounding the Achilles tendon. Instead, a paratenon forms an elastic sleeve around the tendon to permit gliding. It is composed of sheets of dense connective tissue that separate the tendon from the deep fascia of the leg. Within this tendon lie numerous blood vessels and nerves. The peritendinous structure and the abundance of mucopolysaccharides within the sheath permits sliding of the tendon along the adjacent tissues. Proximally, the paratenon is continuous with the muscle fascia and distally it blends with the periosteum of the calcaneus.

HISTOLOGIC ANATOMY

Like most tendons, the Achilles tendon is composed of paralleled bundles of Type 1 collagen.[1] Collagen fibers average 60 μm in diameter. These fibers are organized into fibrils that range from 30 to 130 nm in diameter and assume a wavy pattern. Microfibrils are grouped into fibrils; fibrils are organized into fibers. A group of fibers is organized into fascicles, which are further grouped into bundles. Individual fibrils do not run the entire length of the tendon but rather are linked in succession, necessitating the transfer of stress between associated fibril units.[1] Within the midsubstance of the tendon are fibroblasts that are arranged in longitudinal rows.

Around each collagen bundle is an endotenon, an elastin-rich connective tissue envelope that maintains the bundle's integrity and permits independent bundle gliding in relation to other bundles. This endotenon contains vessels, lymphatics, and nerves. Surrounding the entire gross tendon lies a fine connective tissue sheath called the epitenon with mesotenon and paratenon overlying it.

In a study performed by Cutts,[4] cadaveric observation showed that sarcomere lengths for the muscles in the lower limb vary significantly. The length of soleus sarcomeres averaged 2.033 mm when in anatomic position, and ranged from 1.260 mm in its theoretic shortest position to 3.359 mm in its theoretic longest position. Soleus fibers are shorter Type I fibers and are involved in slow contractures and balance. As for the gastrocnemius muscle, its observed sarcomeres averaged 2.033 mm in length with a range from 1.012 mm at its theoretic shortest position to 4.413 mm at its longest position. Gastrocnemius Type II muscle fibers are responsible for explosive contractures of jumping and running. These sarcomeres are arranged in series, averaging 17,400 before forming the Achilles tendon.

As previously described, the soleus is a pennate muscle. Muscle fibers are arranged anterior to posterior, proximal to distal with an average pennation angle of 19.3°. This is similar to reported findings from Alexander and Vernon[5] that found a mean pennation angle of 20°. Wickiewicz and colleagues[6] described a small portion of highly (60°) pennated fibers along the ventral surface of the muscle.

The gastrocnemius is not regarded as a pennate muscle; however, the individual heads exhibit pennation in relation to one another. Cutts[4] found an average pennation angle of 10.7° of the lateral head. This lends to observations made by Wickiewicz and colleagues[6] that describe the lateral head of the gastrocnemius to be shorter than its medial counterpart, whereas individual fibers are 46% longer in the lateral head compared with the medial, and fibers of the lateral head have a smaller angle of pennation.

BLOOD SUPPLY AND HEMODYNAMICS

As with any tissue, the quality and quantity of vascularization directly affects a tissue's response to trauma and provides the basis for healing. The blood supply to the gastrocnemius and the soleus muscles is usually discussed in 3 separate regions: the musculotendinous junction, direct supply to the tendon, and the tendon-bone junction. Blood vessels from these regions originate from the perimysium, mesotenon-paratenon structure, and periosteum. At the musculotendinous junction, blood is supplied via superficial vessels from surrounding tissues. The main blood supply to the midsubstance of the tendon flows via the paratenon. Vessels within this connective tissue envelope run transversely toward the tendon on its anterior aspect, branch, and then continue longitudinally with the course of the tendon. The blood supply arises from the mesotenon on the anterior aspect of the tendon where the paratenon meets itself. The recurrent branch of the posterior tibial artery supplies the proximal aspect of the tendon, whereas the distal tendon is supplied by the rete arteriosum calcaneare, fibular, and posterior tibial arteries. Vessels enter the tendon at the endotenon, and arterioles continue as capillaries that loop into venules without penetrating collagen bundles. Vessels that supply the bone-tendon junction also supply the lower third of the tendon. These vessels indirectly anastomose with vessels supplying the midsubstance of the tendon.[1,2]

The most commonly cited understanding of the Achilles tendon blood flow is based on cadaveric anatomic research done in the 1950s.[7] We have come to regard the midsubstance of the Achilles as relatively ischemic based on this historic cadaveric research. In 1958, a "watershed" area was identified in the midsubstance of the Achilles tendon through cadaveric injection and analysis of the Achilles peritendinous vessels.[7] It is this "watershed" that has been proposed as the etiology of an ischemic zone in the tendon and proposed a main determinant in weakness and rupture. The term watershed is a geographic concept identifying the point at which 2 bodies of water come together from 2 different directions, or a central zone of land that divides areas drained by different river systems. Indeed, the Achilles tendon has been shown to have multiple sources of blood supply originating distal, proximal, and from the peritendinous structures[7,8] The question is, however, does this anatomic distribution of vessels within the tendon tissues cause a true hemodynamic compromise or ischemia. As early as 1958, Hastad[9] tested the hemodynamic flow in the tendon using a sodium washout technique and noted uniform blood flow throughout the tendon, which challenges the watershed-based ischemia theory. Astrom and colleagues[10] in 1994 used laser Doppler flow analysis to assess real-time tendon circulation in 28 healthy volunteers. They tested the subjects with the Doppler probe inserted into the tendon and assessed hemodynamic flow at rest, during calf muscle contracture and after vascular occlusion. Their findings showed pulsatile flow synchronous with the heart rate evenly distributed throughout the tendon with only a slight decrease at the tendon insertion at the calcaneus.[11] This research challenges the anatomic-based ischemic theory put forth by Lagergren and colleagues.[7] Further hemodynamic research in live subjects has further strengthened the notion that blood flow is uniform throughout the tendon, including the watershed zone.[10,12] Other research has shown an increase in blood flow in the tendon with exercise. Langberg and colleagues[12] used Xe flow measurements to identify a fourfold increase in tendon blood flow 5 cm from the Achilles insertion during exercise. Boushel and colleagues[13] noted that both muscle tendon blood flow increased concurrently with exercise without abnormal shunting of blood.[14] Kubo and colleagues[15] reported both blood volume and oxygen saturation after repetitive muscle contracture did not change.[16] In 2015, Kubo[14] then found that although oxygen consumption did not change when comparing eccentric to concentric muscle contraction, inflow of blood to the tendon was significantly greater during eccentric compared with concentric contractions.

It has been suggested based on work by Cummins and Anson[11] in 1946 that the twisting of the Achilles tendon fibers distally is a possible cause of the purported ischemia of the midsubstance of the tendon. This so called "wringing out" of the tendon, as it has been described by many, is based on these anatomic observations. Although this an attractive circumstantial piece of evidence, the effect of this fiber twisting on real-time blood flow in living tissue has not been confirmed through experimentation. The studies that have shown uniform blood flow throughout the tendon at rest, with contracture and exercise noted previously, would argue against this effect. Further research is needed to make the causal connection between the tendon spatial anatomy (twisting) and the blood flow within the tendon at all levels. Many observations in medicine lead to theories regarding the role that an observation has for function. When these observations are connected with theories that have a strong component of "common sense" or appear on the surface to fit nicely with what we already have learned, the idea begins to be accepted as true through a process of repeated quoting and testing despite lack of true proof. As clinicians and researchers, we must take care not to perpetuate ideas that have not been tested to prove a connection between anatomic observations and theoretic application to physiologic function.

BIOMECHANICS

The gastrocnemius and the soleus act together as the main plantar flexors of the foot at the ankle joint during gait. They are both active during the latter 80% of the stance phase of gait and have a major role in propulsion and balance. The posterior muscles, especially the soleus, act as stabilizers and play a critical role in balance by resisting the ground reactive force on the stance leg as the swing phase extremity moves forward, creating a dorsiflexory moment at the ankle joint. Stabilization forces are converted to push-off force in the stance-phase foot beginning at the point in the gait cycle just after maximal ankle dorsiflexion is achieved with the tibia moving forward producing ankle plantarflexion. The posterior muscle group is inactive just after toe-off and throughout swing. Conditions that result in weakness of the gastrocsoleus unit result in significant imbalance and alterations of the normal gait. Lack of the stabilizing function of the superficial posterior muscles prevents the person from resisting the forces generated from the center of gravity anterior to the knee, which is present in normal gait and results in the person having a tendency to fall forward. In addition, weakness results in compensation with increased activity of the deep posterior muscle group (flexor substitution), which may lead to a variety of foot and digital deformations. Equinus or lack of adequate ankle dorsiflexion in gait can lead to compensation through pronation of the foot. It has been recognized that this effect of compensation for a lack of ankle dorsiflexion can lead to repetitive stress issues in the foot, such as plantar faciosis and forefoot pain. This will be discussed in subsequent articles. Depending on the position of the Achilles tendon relative to the subtalar joint axis, the triceps surae may be a relative supinator or pronator of the subtalar joint. This function will vary depending on foot position and on segmental leg alignment. A more lateral relative position contributes to pronation and more medial position contributes to supination. The position of the tendon insertion can be altered during surgical procedures and thereby change the relative contribution of the gastrocsoleus unit on pronation or supination of the foot.

Because it crosses the knee joint, the gastrocnemius is also a contributor to knee flexion. The contribution of each muscle to plantarflexion power at the ankle has been studied. Silver and colleagues[17] suggested that the soleus is the main plantarflexor at the ankle during normal gait. They showed the soleus to exert nearly double the plantarflexion force at the ankle compared with the gastrocnemius.[17] The medial and lateral heads of the gastrocnemius have the same overall plantarflexion function but have different degrees of contribution, with the medial gastrocnemius head providing more than 70% of the muscle force. Force through the Achilles tendon during exercise can approach 12 times body weight, making the Achilles vulnerable to repetitive stress injury.[18] Late in the stance phase just before heel lift (60%–88%), the knee is in maximal extension and the ankle is in dorsiflexion.[19] This is the point at which the gastrocsoleus is subjected to the maximal stretching force, and therefore there is increased incidence of foot and ankle compensations causing potential symptoms and pathology.[20]

The size and unique structure of the Achilles tendon allow it to function under high loads. In the case of many of the acute and chronic clinical conditions that are discussed in this issue, it is these high forces coupled with structural abnormalities of the foot, ankle, and lower leg that are contributory factors in problems such as mid-substance tendinosis and degeneration. The stress-strain resistance properties of the Achilles are similar to all tendons, with physiologic collagen fiber stretching occurring from 2% to 4% stretch length, microscopic fibril failure at 6% to 8% stretch, and macroscopic failure beyond 8% stretch. Below the failure points of the stress-strain curve, the tendon fibers have the elastic capability to rebound and release energy that is valuable in function.[21] A variety of abnormalities, deformities, and activities can place loads on the tendon that are beyond its capacity to rebound and result in internal tendon fiber damage and degeneration. In contrast to injury, subrupture force application through the tendon is necessary for biochemical signaling of fibroblasts to produce collagen for normal tendon health and to heal injury.[22] This mechanical stress is a necessary component of prevention and recovery from injury and has been shown to increase recovered tendon strength. These principles highlight the importance of continued activity during recovery, with both tendon movement and controlled stress being necessary to promote proper healing. These principles will be applied in other sections in which the detriments of prolonged immobilization and the benefits of movement and controlled force are highlighted as necessary components of tendon recovery.

ACKNOWLEDGMENTS

The author acknowledges the contribution of Jason Weslosky, BS, College of Podiatric Medicine and Surgery, Des Moines University, in the subject research and in assistance writing this article.

REFERENCES

1. Benjamin M, Theobald P, Suzuki D, et al. The anatomy of the Achilles tendon. In: Maffulli N, Almekinders L, editors. The Achilles tendon. London: Springer-Verlag; 2007. p. 5–16.
2. O'Brien M. The anatomy of the Achilles tendon. Foot Ankle Clin 2005;10(2): 225–38 [Review].
3. Ahmed IM, Lagopoulos M, McConnell P, et al. Blood supply of the Achilles tendon. J Orthop Res 1998;16:591–6.
4. Cutts A. The range of sarcomere lengths in the muscles of the human lower limb. J Anat 1988;160:79–88.
5. Alexander RM, Vernon A. The dimensions of the knee and ankle muscles and the forces they exert. J Hum Mov Stud 1975;1:115–23.
6. Wickiewicz TL, Roy RR, Powell PL, et al. Muscle architecture of the human lower limb. Clin Orthop Relat Res 1983;179:275–83.
7. Lagergren C, Lindbom A, Soderberg G. Hypervascularization in chronic inflammation demonstrated by angiography; angiographic, histopathologic, and micro-angiographic studies. Acta Radiol 1958;49(6):441–52.
8. Carr AJ, Norris SH. The blood supply of the calcaneal tendon. J Bone Joint Surg Br 1989;71(1):100–1.
9. Hastad K, Larson L, Lindholm A. Clearance of radiosodium after local deposit in the Achilles tendon. Acta Chir Scand 1958;116:251–5.
10. Aström M, Westlin N. Blood flow in the human Achilles tendon assessed by laser Doppler flowmetry. J Orthop Res 1994;12(2):246–52.

11. Cummins EJ, Anson BJ. The structure of the calcaneal tendon (of Achilles) in relation to orthopedic surgery, with additional observations on the plantaris muscle. Surg Gynecol Obstet 1946;83:107–16.
12. Langberg H, Bülow J, Kjaer M. Blood flow in the peritendinous space of the human Achilles tendon during exercise. Acta Physiol Scand 1998;163(2):149–53.
13. Boushel R, Langberg H, Green S, et al. Blood flow and oxygenation in peritendinous tissue and calf muscle during dynamic exercise in humans. J Physiol 2000; 524(1):305–13.
14. Aström M. Laser Doppler flowmetry in the assessment of tendon blood flow. Scand J Med Sci Sports 2000;10(6):365–7.
15. Kubo K, Ikebukuro T, Tsunoda N, et al. Noninvasive measures of blood volume and oxygen saturation of human Achilles tendon by red laser lights. Acta Physiol (Oxf) 2008;193(3):257–64.
16. Langberg H, Olesen J, Skovgaard D, et al. Age related blood flow around the Achilles tendon during exercise in humans. Eur J Appl Physiol 2001;84(3):246–8.
17. Silver RL, de la Garza J, Rang M. The myth of muscle balance. A study of relative strengths and excursions of normal muscles about the foot and ankle. J Bone Joint Surg Br 1985;67(3):432–7.
18. Benjamin M, Toumi H, Ralphs JR, et al. Where tendons and ligaments meet bone: attachment sites ('entheses') in relation to exercise and/or mechanical load. J Anat 2006;208(4):471–90 [Review].
19. Cappozzo A, Leo T, Pedotti A. A general computing method for the analysis of human locomotion. J Biomech 1975;8(5):307–20.
20. Cazeau C, Stiglitz Y. Effects of gastrocnemius tightness on forefoot during gait. Foot Ankle Clin 2014;19(4):649–57 [Review].
21. Wang JH. Mechanobiology of tendon. J Biomech 2006;39(9):1563–82 [Review].
22. Eliasson P, Andersson T, Hammerman M, et al. Primary gene response to mechanical loading in healing rat Achilles tendons. J Appl Physiol (1985) 2013; 114(11):1519–26.

Imaging Techniques and Indications

 CrossMark

James M. Mahoney, DPM

KEYWORDS

- Tendinopathy • Radiograph • Ultrasonography • MRI

KEY POINTS

- Although not the preferred imaging method, radiographs are able to detect subtle pathologic changes to the Achilles tendon and neighboring structures.
- Ultrasonography imaging is the modality of choice for diagnosing focal Achilles tendon disease and differentiating partial from complete tears.
- Advanced imaging studies, including ultrasonography, are unnecessary and do not improve patient care.
- Most Achilles disorders can be diagnosed clinically without the need for imaging.

 Video content accompanies this article at http://www.podiatric.theclinics.com.

INTRODUCTION

In this article, tendinopathy is used to describe the clinical picture of pain, swelling, and decreased activity that accompanies overuse injuries to the Achilles tendon, including the body of the tendon and the paratenon.[1] The disorders are further divided into noninsertional, which include Achilles tendon rupture, and insertional, including enthesopathy. The terms acute and chronic as a means to distinguish the imaging characteristics of Achilles disorders are avoided because the time frames are arbitrary and not based on clinical or histopathologic findings.[2] The radiographic, ultrasonographic, and MRI characteristics that can be used for establishing a diagnosis of tendinopathy are discussed, as well as their benefits and limitations.

ANATOMIC CONSIDERATIONS

From posterior to anterior, the posterior soft tissue structures of the ankle are arranged in the following order: retrocalcaneal (adventitious) bursa, Achilles tendon, anatomic bursa, Kager triangle, and the flexor hallucis longus muscle belly.

College of Podiatric Medicine and Surgery, Des Moines University, 3200 Grand Avenue, Des Moines, IA 50312, USA
E-mail address: James.Mahoney@dmu.edu

Clin Podiatr Med Surg 34 (2017) 115–128
http://dx.doi.org/10.1016/j.cpm.2016.10.014
0891-8422/17/© 2016 Elsevier Inc. All rights reserved.

The retrocalcaneal bursa, which lies between the skin and tendon, is inconsistently found and secondary to inflammation, usually caused by pressure from the heel counter of a shoe. There is a natural twist to the fibers of the tendon, such that the medial fibers proximally become posterior at its insertion into the calcaneus. This twist causes tension in the tendon, which is greatest at 2 to 6 cm above the insertion.[3] Most anatomic studies show that this area is also hypovascular, and is often called a water-shed region.[3] Investigators often cite this as the cause for noninsertional injuries. Kvist[4] found that, in competitive athletes, noninsertional disorder occurred 66% of the time, and insertional 23% to 25%. The remainder occurred at the myotendinous junction. However, Ahmed and colleagues'[5] histologic analysis showed that the entire length of the tendon has a poor blood supply that does not vary significantly along its length. Furthermore, the smallest cross-sectional area, and therefore the greatest area of tension, was found at the 2-c to 6-cm region proximal to the insertion, suggesting that the blood supply may not be an important factor in Achilles rupture.

The paratenon surrounds the entire length of the Achilles and forms a thin space between the tendon and the crural fascia.[2] The anatomic bursa lies between the posterior-superior surface of the calcaneus and the anterior border of the tendon. Disorder in the Achilles can lead to inflammation of this bursa, as well as the retrocalcaneal bursa.[2] It can also cause changes to the Kager triangle, which is the fatty tissue space that lies between the anterior surface of the Achilles with which it forms a sharp interface, the superior surface of the calcaneus, and the posterior surface of the muscle of flexor hallucis longus.[6] Theobald and colleagues[7] showed that the flexor hallucis longus part moves the bursal wedge during plantarflexion, the Achilles part protects the blood vessels entering the tendon, and the bursal wedge portion minimizes pressure changes in the anatomic bursa.

CONVENTIONAL RADIOGRAPHY

Most clinicians do not consider a radiograph as a tool for diagnosing Achilles tendon disorder because it lacks soft tissue contrast. However, it is inexpensive, easy to administer, and fast, and it may lead to valuable diagnostic information. It is best to use a high-contrast (low-kilovolt) technique, otherwise the changes may be subtle and difficult to find.[6]

The normal Achilles tendon should be no more than 8 mm in the anterior-posterior dimension, being thicker proximally and tapering only slightly into its calcaneal insertion (**Fig. 1**).[6] Tendinopathy leads to a thickening of the tendon, as well as blurring of

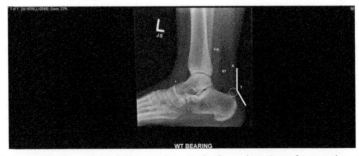

Fig. 1. Radiograph of normal Achilles tendon. Circle shows location of retrocalcaneal bursa. A, Achilles tendon; FHL, flexor hallucis longus muscle; KT, Kager triangle; T, Toygar angle (>150°); WT, weight.

the interface between the Achilles and Kager triangle.[6] The anterior border of a thickened tendon may bow into the triangle causing a convex appearance to the tendon. The normal anatomic bursa is seen as a radiolucent interval about 2 to 3 mm in length that extends between the anterior border of the tendon and the superior-posterior surface of the calcaneus.[6] Its absence suggests inflammation of either the bursa and/or the Achilles (**Fig. 2**).

Bony erosions within the posterior-superior surface of the calcaneus, in the vicinity of the anatomic bursa, strongly suggest an enthesopathy related to an inflammatory arthritis (**Fig. 3**).[8] Because these diseases attack the synovium, the bursal lining adjacent to the calcaneus is affected and can secondarily erode the adjacent surface of the calcaneus. Spur formation within the Achilles tendon is common at its insertion and can develop without inflammation or microtrauma (**Fig. 4**). This finding suggests an adaptational process in response to increased mechanical stress at the bone-tendon interface.[9]

In a frank rupture of the tendon, the Kager triangle loses its sharp margins and also becomes smaller and more radio-opaque.[10] The Toygar angle, formed by the angle of the posterior skin surface overlying the Achilles, decreases to less than 150°,[11] which was found to occur 12% of the time.[10] There is often a positive Arner sign where the anterior surface of the Achilles curves away from the calcaneus between its insertion and the upper part of calcaneus (**Fig. 5**),[11] and this occurred 48% of the time in Cetti's[10] study. The anterior-posterior width of the tendon would also be expected to be greater than 8 mm. Overall, the accuracy of predicting the rupture site on radiographs is not good, with 58% of patients having surgical verification of the tear within 10 mm of the interpretation on radiograph.[10]

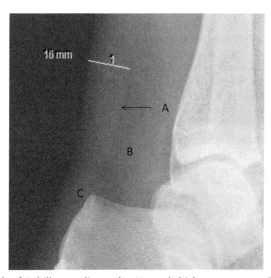

Fig. 2. Radiograph of Achilles tendinopathy. Normal thickness averages 8 mm in the anteroposterior direction. 1 shows a 16 mm thickness of the Achilles tendon. A, arrow is pointing to the anterior bowing of Achilles into Kager triangle; B, increased opacity of Kager triangle; C, retrocalcaneal bursitis as seen by lack of radiolucency between posterior heel and Achilles tendon. (*Courtesy of* Brooke Army Medical Center, San Antonio, TX; with permission.)

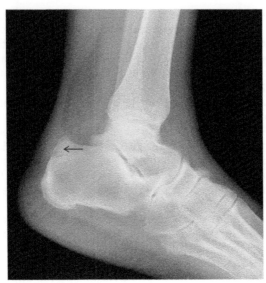

Fig. 3. Radiograph of Achilles enthesopathy secondary to rheumatoid arthritis. Note the erosions on the posterior-superior aspect of the calcaneus (*arrow*) and thickened Achilles tendon at its insertion. (*Courtesy of* Brooke Army Medical Center, San Antonio, TX; with permission.)

ULTRASONOGRAPHY

Because of its accessibility, large tissue volume, and fairly straight course, the Achilles tendon is ideal for imaging with musculoskeletal ultrasonography. It also allows easy contralateral assessment and dynamic evaluation through active and passive ankle motion. Unlike conventional radiography, it does not use ionizing radiation. It carries a high positive predictive value for Achilles tendinopathy.[2]

Imaging with ultrasonography is performed in both the longitudinal and transverse orientations (**Fig. 6**). When viewed with a high-frequency transducer longitudinally (>7.5 MHz), the normal Achilles reveals parallel echogenic lines, which represent the fascicles of the tendon, and when viewed transversely the fascicles appear either as echogenic lines or points (**Fig. 7**).[12] Because the tendon is so close to the skin surface, it is best to use a 15-MHz transducer,[6] which provides the best spatial resolution and clearest image.[13] In addition, using a microlinear transducer whose shape resembles a hockey stick allows easy placement of the transducer (**Fig. 8**).[13] On transverse images, the anterior-posterior diameter of the Achilles is normally 4 to 6 mm.[6] The

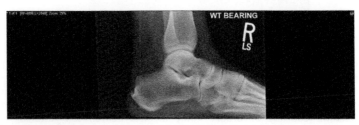

Fig. 4. Radiograph showing calcification of Achilles tendon insertion.

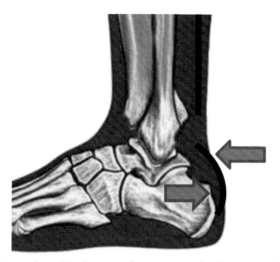

Fig. 5. Positive Arner sign. Distal arrow shows a completely ruptured Achilles tendon curving away from its insertion on the posterior calcaneus; proximal arrow shows curving of completely ruptured Achilles tendon anteriorly at its point of rupture.

Kager triangle shows mottled hypoechogenicity compared with the echogenic tendon.[6] The retrocalcaneal bursa may contain up to 3 mm of fluid, whereas the adventitious bursa usually has no fluid.[14]

Tendinopathy occurs most commonly on the posterior-medial portion in the mid-portion of the Achilles.[15] Tendinopathy typically shows abnormal thickening of tendon beyond 8 mm, areas of hypoechogenicity within the tendon, and neovascularity with color and power Doppler (**Fig. 9**).[6] Color Doppler superimposes color on the gray-scale sonogram and indicates the speed and direction of flow. Red indicates blood flow toward the transducer, and blue indicates flow away from the transducer. Power Doppler displays the strength of the flow in color, but not the speed and direction. The stronger the signal, the whiter it appears. It is 3 times stronger than color Doppler and detects smaller and lower-velocity vessels.[16]

Neovascularity was first described by Alfredson[17] and it is an abnormal finding. He suggests that the ingrowth of vessels and nerves into the damaged tendon are the source of pain. Eccentric stretching then damages the vessels and nerves, which makes them disappear and is consistent with healing. Color and power Doppler so-nography resulted in a specificity of 100% and a sensitivity of 50% for symptomatic Achilles tendinopathy.[18] However, de Vos and colleagues[19] showed that neovessels were found in only 63% of symptomatic tendons, were not associated with clinical severity, and their presence or absence was not associated with a better or worse outcome at 3 months.

Partial tears can be difficult to distinguish from thickening of the Achilles in noninser-tional tendinopathy.[6] However, one study showed that partial tears were more commonly seen with intratendinous disorders and greater than 10-mm thickness in the anterior-posterior diameter.[20] Unlike partial tears, full tears are easily identifiable.[21] Paavola and colleagues[21] correctly identified 25 out of 26 full tears before surgery. Ul-trasonography has been found to have a sensitivity of 100%, a specificity of 83%, and an accuracy of 92% in diagnosing complete tears.[22] Full-thickness tears often show nonpalpable tendon at the site of injury, tendon retraction, and a posterior acoustic

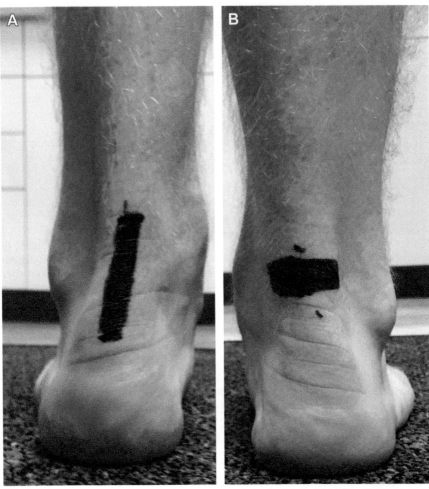

Fig. 6. Orientation of ultrasonography transducer for Achilles tendon. (*A*) Longitudinal. (*B*) Transverse. (*Courtesy of* James Renier, BS, Des Moines University, Des Moines, IA.)

shadowing at the tear site.[22] Clinicians must be careful not to confuse the intact plantaris tendon along the medial aspect of the Achilles with a severe partial tear.[6] Examiners can also perform dynamic ankle movement, which could help differentiate partial-thickness from full-thickness tears, as well as guide surgical planning (Videos 1 and 2).[6] Full tears are missed 20% of the time by providers.[2]

Insertional Achilles tendinopathy often shows calcifications within the body of the tendon. Calcifications are hyperechoic and show posterior acoustic shadowing.[23] Posterior acoustic shadowing is seen as hypoechoic or anechoic areas that extend below the calcification (**Fig. 10**).[13]

Paratenonitis can be identified as a thickening of the hypoechoic paratenon great than 1.27 mm.[24]

The size and shape of the retrocalcaneal and adventitious bursae change with ankle dorsiflexion and plantarflexion. Distention of the retrocalcaneal bursa greater than 3 mm in the anterior-posterior direction is abnormal.[23]

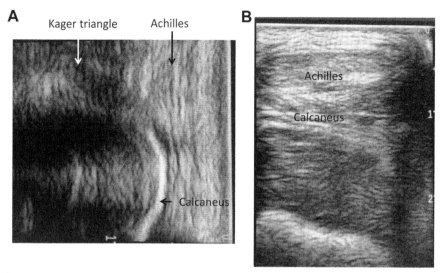

Fig. 7. Normal Achilles tendon in longitudinal (*A*) and transverse (*B*) orientation. (*Courtesy of* James Renier, Des Moines, IA.)

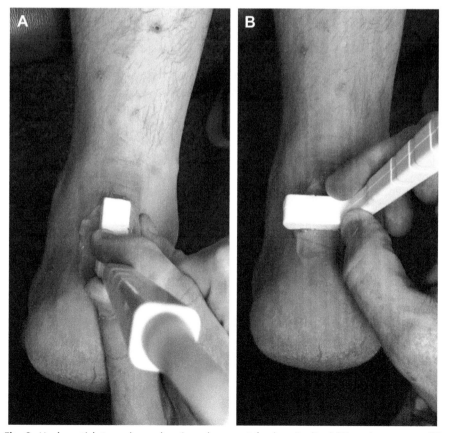

Fig. 8. Hockey-stick transducer showing placement for longitudinal (*A*) and transverse (*B*) images. (*Courtesy of* James Renier, Des Moines, IA.)

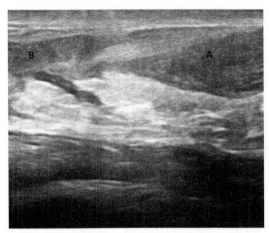

Fig. 9. Tendinopathy of Achilles tendon in longitudinal axis. A and B comprise the width of Achilles tendon. A, overt tendinopathy; B, less damaged fibers. (*Courtesy of* Nathan H. Schwartz, DPM, Smyrna, GA.)

Sonoelastography is a fairly new form of ultrasonography that aids in the diagnosis of disorders that are not evident on routine ultrasonography examination. It evaluates tissue elasticity, with painful tendons showing increased stiffness compared with normal tendons.[2] The technique produces an elastogram on which blue, red, and yellow-green colors suggest hard, soft, and intermediate tissue stiffness, respectively.[25] Galetti and colleagues[25] showed that, out of 35 patients with Achilles tendon pain who were negative for disorder on routine ultrasonography, 27 had positive findings on sonoelastography.

MRI

The normal Achilles tendon is hypointense on all MRI sequences because of its low mobile water content.[2] It averages 6 mm in thickness and is normally thicker in tall patients, men, and the elderly.[26] On axial images, the anterior margin is concave and the

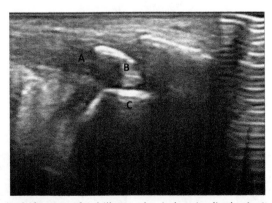

Fig. 10. Insertional calcification of Achilles tendon in longitudinal axis. A, damaged Achilles tendon; B, calcifications within Achilles tendon; C, calcaneus. (*Courtesy of* Nathan H. Schwartz, DPM, Smyrna, GA.)

anterior and posterior margins are parallel below the soleus attachment on sagittal images, and on coronal sections the sides are straight.[26] Small, punctate areas of high signal are often seen distally, especially on the axial images, and represent normal interfascicular membranes (**Fig. 11**).[26] Normal retrocalcaneal bursae average 1 mm in the anterior-posterior dimension, 6 mm in the transverse dimension, and 3 mm superior to inferior.[27] Intravenous contrast is not used routinely; however, it may be used to aid in the diagnosis of bursitis (**Fig. 12**).[28]

Increased thickness, a fusiform shape, and increased signal on T1, T2, and short tau inversion recovery (STIR) images strongly suggests Achilles tendinopathy (**Fig. 13**).[2] Intratendinous hyperintensity usually represents partial tearing, fiber disruption, or mucoid degeneration.[2] It is necessary to differentiate the hyperintensity of intratendinous disorder from the hyperintensity seen with the so-called magic-angle artifact. This artifact usually occurs in the tendon where the fibers are normally twisted so that, on a T1 image, there is increased signal intensity within the tendon that suggests disorder, but on T2 the tendon appears normal.[28] By using a formula that measured tendon depth, the length of the retrocalcaneal bursa, and the area of tendon, Weber and colleagues[29] showed a sensitivity of 97% and a specificity of 91% for differentiating between normal and diseased tendons.

Paratenonitis shows a halo of hyperintensity on T2 and STIR images and may extend into the subcutaneous fat posteriorly and into the Kager triangle anteriorly.[30] Insertional tendonitis shows distal thickening with ill-defined high signal that can resemble a partial tear. Any calcifications present within the insertional area usually have a normal marrow signal[28] and represent dystrophic changes.[26] This calcification may progress to ossification that shows cortical bone and trabeculae and probably represents a different degenerative pathway from calcification.[26] Inflammatory enthesopathies, such as Reiter disease, may manifest with erosive changes in the posterior-superior aspect of the calcaneus and represent adjacent synovitis of the overlying retrocalcaneal bursa.[30]

Partial and complete tears have high signal on T2 and the edges are retracted from each other, probably with atrophy of the tendon at the edges (**Fig. 14**).[26]

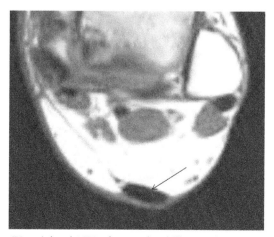

Fig. 11. Transverse T1-weighted MRI of normal Achilles tendon. Arrow points to normal areas of hyperintensity within the tendon, representing interfascicular membranes. (*Courtesy of* Paul Dayton, DPM, MS, FACFAS, Fort Dodge, IA.)

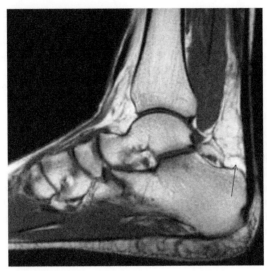

Fig. 12. Sagittal T2-weighted MRI of retrocalcaneal bursitis (*arrow*) showing enlargement and hyperintensity. (*Courtesy of* Paul Dayton, DPM, MS, FACFAS, Fort Dodge, IA.)

ECONOMICS OF USE

When using advanced imaging for Achilles tendon disorders, ultrasonography is the modality of choice for diagnosing focal tendon disease and differentiating partial from complete tears.[31] It also is less expensive. When reviewing data from the Centers

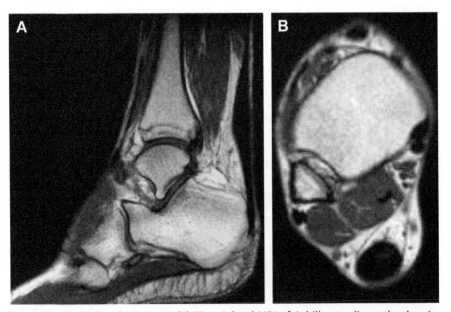

Fig. 13. Sagittal (*A*) and transverse (*B*) T2-weighted MRI of Achilles tendinopathy showing thickening and central hyperintensity suggesting mucoid degeneration. (*Courtesy of* Paul Dayton, DPM, MS, FACFAS, Fort Dodge, IA.)

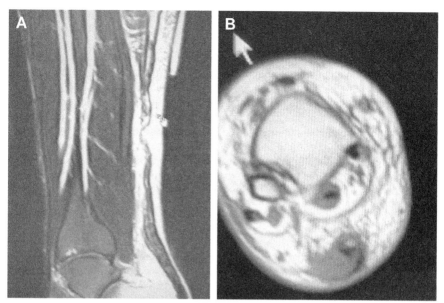

Fig. 14. Sagittal STIR (*A*) and transverse T1-weighted MRI (*B*) of complete tear of Achilles tendon. (*Courtesy of* Paul Dayton, DPM, MS, FACFAS, Fort Dodge, IA.)

for Medicare and Medicaid Services, CPT (Current Procedural Terminology) code 73721 (MRI of lower extremity without contrast), the professional component was about $75.00 and the technical component around $180.00.[32] Compare this with CPT code 76,881 (ultrasound extremity, nonvascular, complete) for which the professional and technical components are $35.00 and $90.00, respectively, and the benefits to the US health care system can be seen.[32] Parker and colleagues[33] projected that costs for musculoskeletal imaging in 2020 will be $3.6 billion, of which $2.0 billion will be for MRI. By evaluating more than 3600 MRI reports from 1996 to 2005, they determined that 45% of primary diagnoses and 31% of all diagnoses could have been made with ultrasonography, resulting in substantial cost savings.

However, there is broad agreement in the literature that a substantial amount of advanced imaging studies, including ultrasonography, are unnecessary and do not improve patient care.[34] The investigators cite several factors that contribute to this overuse, including that the evidence for using advanced imaging is incomplete and that advertising causes patients to pressure their physicians to use the new modalities without any thought to risks and costs. Also, self-referral by physicians who own advanced imaging modalities causes a significant increase in imaging use. There is also a liability risk, and lawsuits arising from overuse of testing are very rare. In addition, medical training encourages students and residents to use every tool available to arrive at a diagnosis.

In particular, there is overwhelming consensus that most Achilles disorders can be diagnosed clinically without the need for imaging.[35] Garras and colleagues[36] go so far as to conclude that physical examination is more sensitive than MRI in diagnosing complete tendon ruptures. In their study, the clinical signs of a positive Thompson test, a positive Matles test or decreased ankle resting tension compared with the contralateral side (less than 20°–30° of ankle plantarflexion with the patient prone and the knee at 90°), and a palpable defect predicted a complete tear 100% of the time, whereas MRI sensitivity was 91% compared with intraoperative findings. Imaging is of most benefit for confounding diagnoses or trying to differentiate partial from complete Achilles tears.[30]

When comparing ultrasonography with MRI analysis of symptomatic tendons, Khan and colleagues[37] identified disorder in 65% of symptomatic tendons and normal morphology in 68% of asymptomatic tendons on ultrasonography, and disorder in 56% of symptomatic tendons and normal morphology in 94% of asymptomatic tendons on MRI. Furthermore, the addition of color and power Doppler did not improve the diagnostic ability of ultrasonography. They concluded that imaging tests should be ordered judiciously because there is a high number of false-positive and false-negative diagnoses. They further suggest that ultrasonography and MRI might be of more use when patients fail conservative care for Achilles tendinopathy or for inexperienced clinicians.

SUMMARY

Achilles tendon disorder is, for the most part, readily identifiable on most imaging techniques. However, the available evidence suggests that clinical examination is often the best tool to use for diagnosis, and that MRI and ultrasonography are often unnecessary and should be considered only when the diagnosis is confounding or a patient does not respond to recommended conservative care. Clinical decision-making tools should be developed that predict when advanced imaging techniques should be used in the evaluation of Achilles tendon disorder.

SUPPLEMENTARY DATA

Supplementary data related to this article can be found online at http://dx.doi.org/10.1016/j.cpm.2016.10.014.

REFERENCES

1. Jarvinen TA, Kannus P, Paavola M, et al. Achilles tendon injuries. Curr Opin Rheumatol 2001;13:150–5.
2. Wijesekera NT, Calder JD, Lee JC. Imaging in the assessment and management of Achilles tendinopathy and paratendinitis. Semin Musculoskelet Radiol 2011;15: 89–100.
3. Chen TM, Rozen WM, Pan W, et al. The arterial anatomy of the Achilles tendon: anatomical study and clinical implications. Clin Anat 2009;22:377–85.
4. Kvist M. Achilles tendon injuries in athletes. Ann Chir Gynaecol 1991;80:188–201.
5. Ahmed IM, Lagopoulos M, McConnell P, et al. Blood supply of the Achilles tendon. J Orthop Res 1998;16:591–6.
6. Bleakney RR, White LM, Maffulli N. Imaging of the Achilles tendon. In: Maffulli N, Almekinders LC, editors. The Achilles tendon. New York: Springer Publishing Co; 2007. p. 25–38.
7. Theobald P, Bydder G, Dent C, et al. The functional anatomy of Kager's fat pad in relation to retrocalcaneal problems and other hindfoot disorders. J Anat 2006; 208:91–7.
8. Jacobson JA, Girish G, Jiang Y, et al. Radiographic evaluation of arthritis: inflammatory conditions. Radiology 2008;248:378–89.
9. Johansson KJJ, Sarimo JJ, Lempainen LL, et al. Calcific spurs at the insertion of the Achilles tendon: a clinical and histological study. Muscles Ligaments Tendons J 2013;2:273–7.

10. Cetti R, Andersen I. Roentgenographic diagnoses of ruptured Achilles tendons. Clin Orthop Relat Res 1993;286:215–21.
11. Combalia A, Nardi J. Roentgenographic assessment of Achilles tendon rupture. J Accid Emerg Med 1995;12:230–1.
12. Weireb JH, Sheth C, Apostolakos J, et al. Tendon structure, disease, and imaging. Muscles Ligaments Tendons J 2014;4:66–73.
13. Schwartz NH. Ultrasound image optimization. In: Ultrasound of the foot and ankle. New York: McGraw-Hill Education; 2015. p. 9–15.
14. Dong Q, Fessel DP. Achilles tendon ultrasound technique. Am J Roentgenol 2009;193:W173.
15. Counsel P, Comin J, Davenport M, et al. Pattern of fascicular involvement in midportion Achilles tendinopathy at ultrasound. Sports Health 2015;7:424–8.
16. Babcock DS, Patriquin H, LaFortune M, et al. Power Doppler sonography and basic principles and clinical application in children. Pediatr Radiol 1996;26:109–15.
17. Alfredson H. Chronic midportion Achilles tendinopathy: an update on research and treatment. Clin Sports Med 2003;22:727–41.
18. Reiter M, Ulreich N, Dirisamer A, et al. Colour and power Doppler sonography in symptomatic Achilles tendon disease. Int J Sports Med 2004;25:301–5.
19. de Vos R, Weir A, Cobben LPJ, et al. The value of power Doppler ultrasonography in Achilles tendinopathy. Am J Sports Med 2007;35:1696–701.
20. Astrom M, Gentz CF, Nilsson P, et al. Imaging in chronic Achilles tendinopathy: a comparison of ultrasonography, magnetic resonance imaging and surgical findings in 27 histologically verified cases. Skeletal Radiol 1996;25:615–20.
21. Paavola M, Paakkala T, Kannus P, et al. Ultrasonography in the differential diagnosis of Achilles tendon injuries and related disorders: a comparison between pre-operative ultrasonography and surgical findings. Acta Radiol 1998;39:612–9.
22. Hartgerink P, Fessell DP, Jacobson JA, et al. Full- versus partial-thickness Achilles tendon tears: sonographic accuracy and characterization in 26 cases with surgical correlation. Radiology 2001;220:406–12.
23. Fessell DP, van Holsbeeck MT. Foot and ankle sonography. Radiol Clin North Am 1999;37:837–58.
24. Stecco A, Busoni F, Stecco C, et al. Comparative ultrasonographic evaluation of the Achilles paratenon in symptomatic and asymptomatic subjects: an imaging study. Surg Radiol Anat 2015;37:281–5.
25. Galetti S, Oliva F, Masiero S, et al. Sonoelastography in the diagnosis of tendinopathies: an added value. Muscles Ligaments Tendons J 2015;5:325–30.
26. Schweitzer ME, Karasick D. MR imaging of disorders of the Achilles tendon. AJR Am J Roentgenol 2000;175:613–26.
27. Bottger BA, Schweitzer ME, El-Noueam KI, et al. MR imaging of the normal and abnormal retrocalcaneal bursae. Am J Roentgenol 1998;170:1239–41.
28. Pierre-Jerome C, Moncayo V, Terk MR. MRI of the Achilles tendon: a comprehensive review of the anatomy, biomechanics, and imaging of overuse tendinopathies. Acta Radiol 2010;4:438–54.
29. Weber C, Wedegartner U, Maas LC, et al. MR imaging of the Achilles tendon: evaluation of criteria for the differentiation of asymptomatic and symptomatic tendons. Rofo 2011;183:631–40 [in German].
30. Peterson B, Fitzgerald V, Schreibman K. Musculotendinous magnetic resonance imaging of the ankle. Semin Roentgenol 2010;45:250–76.
31. Jacobson JA. Musculoskeletal ultrasound and MRI: which do I choose? Semin Musculoskelet Radiol 2005;9:135–49.

32. Centers for Medicare & Medicaid Services Web site. PFS relative value files. Available at: www.cms.hhs.gov/physician-fee-schedule/PSFRV/list. Accessed May 24, 2016.
33. Parker L, Nazarian LN, Carrino JA, et al. Musculoskeletal imaging: Medicare use, costs, and potential for cost substitution. J Am Coll Radiol 2008;5:182–8.
34. Hillman BJ, Goldsmith JC. The uncritical use of high-tech medical imaging. N Engl J Med 2010;363:4–6.
35. Asplund CA, Best TM. Achilles tendon disorders. BMJ 2013;346:f1262.
36. Garras DN, Raikin SM, Bhat SB, et al. MRI is unnecessary for diagnosing acute Achilles tendon ruptures. Clin Orthop Relat Res 2012;470:2268–73.
37. Khan KM, Forster BB, Robinson J, et al. Are ultrasound and magnetic resonance imaging of value in assessment of Achilles tendon disorders? A two year prospective study. Br J Sports Med 2003;37:149–53.

Noninsertional Achilles Tendinopathy Pathologic Background and Clinical Examination

Mindi Feilmeier, DPM

KEYWORDS

- Achilles • Tendinopathy • Tendinosis

KEY POINTS

- Achilles tendinopathy includes a spectrum of histologic pathologic findings ranging from acute inflammation to chronic degeneration and fiber rupture.
- Tendinopathy is a clinically diagnosed condition with specific clinical cues leading to accurate diagnosis.

INTRODUCTION

The term tendinopathy includes a series of pathologies, all of which have a combination of pain, swelling, and impaired performance.[1] Most authorities advocate the use of the term tendinopathy to encompass each of the subclasses of Achilles tendon pathology. The terms tendinosis, tendinitis, and peritendinitis are all within the main heading of tendinopathy, and this terminology provides a more accurate understanding of the condition and highlights the uniformity of clinical findings while distinguishing the individual histopathological findings of each condition.[2,3] Understanding both the clinical features and the underlying histopathology leads to a more accurate clinical diagnosis and subsequent treatment selection.

This is an important distinction, because the misuse of the term tendinitis in the clinical diagnosis and treatment of these disorders can lead to the underestimation of chronic degenerative nature of many tendinopathies, which may affect the treatment selection.[2] Specifically, treating the chronic degenerative forms of tendinosis with immobilization and anti-inflammatory medications commonly used for acute inflammatory processes may lead to treatment failures and have the potential to drive

Financial Disclosure: The authors have nothing to disclose.
College of Podiatric Medicine and Surgery, Des Moines University, 3200 Grand Avenue, Des Moines, IA 50312, USA
E-mail address: Mindi.Feilmeier@dmu.edu

unnecessary surgery.[4] The treatment of these pathologies, namely noninsertional tendinosis, will be discussed in subsequent articles and is guided by an understanding of the underlying pathologic process.

The basic etiology of the Achilles tendinopathy is known to be multifactorial. The pathophysiology of chronic Achilles tendinopathy is thought to involve the cellular and molecular response to microscopic tearing of the tendon when forces beyond the elastic capabilities of the tendon are applied to the tissues leading to chronic degeneration. Histologic examination of the affected tissue demonstrates an irregular shape and a higher rate of apoptosis.[5–7] Although inflammation occurs around the tendon, biopsies demonstrate no inflammatory cells infiltrating the tendon. Tendinopathy is understood as a failed healing response within the extracellular matrix that is mediated by a cascade of proinflammatory molecules that include interleukin-1B, prostaglandin E2, and nitric oxide.[8,9] In patients who develop tendinopathy, these mediators induce apoptosis, signal pain responses, and increase the production of matrix metalloproteinases (MMPs).[7] This response leads to degeneration of the tendon, rather than signaling a repair process.[8,10]

Histologic evaluation of tissue taken from ruptured Achilles tendons has been shown to contain more degeneration than those taken from patients with tendinopathy and uninvolved controls.[11,12] A similar study revealed that almost all of the Achilles tendons operated on for rupture showed signs of hypoxic degenerative tendinopathy, calcifying tendinopathy, mucoid degeneration, or tendolipamatosis.[13] In a large retrospective case-control study by Tallon and colleagues,[14] no spontaneous Achilles tendon ruptures were found in patients with healthy tendons. It is important to note, however, that Achilles tendon ruptures can take place suddenly without any preceding signs or symptoms.[12]

Because the Achilles tendon is the strongest and thickest tendon in the body and is subjected to unique forces during the activities of living, it is highly subject to tendinopathy, which can ultimately result in chronic degenerative changes, as well as calcification and mucoidlike degeneration, leading to Achilles tendinosis.[12] Because of the unique anatomy of the Achilles tendon, including its rotational change with spiraling proximal to its insertion, the Achilles is under significant biomechanical strain 2 to 6 cm proximal to its insertion into the calcaneus. While the degeneration at this area has been attributed to avascularity, this may not be the case, as discussed in this issue (see Paul Dayton's article, "Anatomic, Vascular, and Mechanical Overview of the Achilles Tendon," in this issue).

As noted previously, several theories exist regarding the etiology of Achilles tendinopathy. These include overuse, poor tissue vascularity, mechanical imbalances of the extremity, and a genetic predisposition.[4,15,16] Tendinopathy secondary to overuse is thought to arise from repetitive microtrauma in the central portion of the tendon. A retrospective case-control study identified several patient factors that were more likely to be associated with Achilles tendinopathy: hypertension, diabetes, obesity, and a previous exposure to steroids or estrogen. Each of these factors has the potential to decrease the microvascularity of tendons and as such have been postulated to play a role in the development of Achilles tendinopathy.[17] Other studies have found advancing age, previous injury, exposure to quinolone antibiotics, and endocrine and metabolic abnormalities to be associated with Achilles tendinopathy.[18–20] From a biomechanical standpoint, Williams and colleagues[21] found patients with Achilles tendinopathy to have decreased tibial external rotation during running, which was attributed to an imbalance of muscle forces in the transverse-plane of motion that increases the strain on the Achilles tendon. Finally, the gene for matrix metalloprotease-3 (MMP-3) is involved in the homeostasis of the ground substance surrounding tendons. Variants in the gene are potential genetic contributions to the development of tendinopathy.[7,22,23]

Vascular ingrowth, known as neovascularization, and neural ingrowth have been associated with Achilles tendinosis as well. Several investigators have reported an increase in tendon thickness, which is associated with clinical symptoms and impaired function, to be accompanied by an increase in neovessels.[8,24–28] Studies have found that after conservative treatment for Achilles tendinopathy as the tendon size decreases, returning to a more normal size, and as function increases, there is an associated decrease in the number of vessels identified at the area by power Doppler.[29] These findings are contrary to previously held beliefs that a decrease in blood flow is a cause of chronic Achilles tendinosis and is an important concept when selecting treatment options.[30]

In a series of patients with Achilles tendinopathy, Alfredson and collegues[31] used a microcatheter and microdialysis to sample the environment within and around the Achilles tendon. Their findings showed no change in the levels of prostaglandin E2, a marker of inflammation, compared with controls. They did find an increase in concentration of glutamate, a neurotransmitter associated with pain.[31] Scott and colleagues[32] demonstrated a statistically higher level of immunoreactivity for vesicular glutamate transporter VGluT2 in tendons with tendinosis compared with normal tendons and that the VGluT2 was expressed by tenocytes. These findings suggest that free glutamate may be produced and released by the tenocytes and this may impact apocrine and paracrine functions that play a role in the development of tendinosis. Several roles that glutamate may play include tenocyte proliferation and apoptosis, as well as extracellular metabolism, nociception, and blood flow.[32]

Others studies have identified that in patients with Achilles tendinopathy there are also higher levels of lactate, increased expression of enzymes producing acetylcholine and catecholamines, increased substance P, and increased neurokinin-1 (NK-1).[31,33–37] All of these substances are hypothesized to contribute to the pathophysiology of tendinopathy. High lactate levels suggest the presence of ischemia or anaerobic conditions within the tendon in Achilles tendinopathy. Acetylcholine has vasoactive, trophic, and pain-modulating effects that could contribute to tendinopathy. Autocrine/paracrine effects between the diseased tenocytes could increase muscularinic receptors on those cells and increase the production of acetylcholine.[35] Substance P has been associated with pain transmission, cell growth, and angiogenesis, and the organization of tendon and NK-1 receptors are the preferred receptor for substance P, therefore interactions between the 2 may influence tendon repair.[36,37] Currently, the specific contributions of these mechanisms to tendinopathy are not understood completely. Further research may prove to identify additional treatment options for this pathology by focusing on these cellular effects.

Achilles tendinopathy is common among athletes, especially those who are active runners.[38] Force through the Achilles tendon during exercise can approach 12 times body weight, making the Achilles vulnerable to repetitive stress injury.[39] Additionally, there may be a contribution of poor training technique, increased mileage, and an imbalance between muscle power and tendon elasticity.[10,40] Late in the stance phase just before heel lift, the knee is in maximal extension and the ankle is in dorsiflexion. This is the point at which the gastrocsoleus is subjected to the maximal stretching force and therefore there is increased incidence of foot and ankle compensations causing potential symptoms and pathology.[41] The high forces of training as well as excessive weight and explosive activities, combined with the unique structure and function of the Achilles can lead to midsubstance tendinosis. When the tendon is placed into a situation in which the chronic load results in continued strain beyond the elastic limits, the collagen fibers are damaged and fail to repair themselves and degeneration ensues.

CLINICAL PRESENTATION

The history of Achilles tendinopathy is often typical, with subjective complaints of pain localized to the Achilles region, typically 2 to 6 cm proximal to the insertion into the calcaneus, and morning stiffness.[42] Patients may complain of noticing increased swelling and/or a "bump" on the back of the Achilles region, although this is not always present. Pain quality can range from sharp, to dull and burning. Oftentimes there is an accompanying increase in activity associated with the symptoms. The differential diagnosis of Achilles tendinopathy includes many pathologies, including retrocalcaneal bursitis, os trigonum, tarsal tunnel syndrome, posterior tibial tendon pathology, arthritic conditions, and stress fracture.[42] The Victorian Institute of Sport Assessment-Achilles (VISA-A) questionnaire is a valid, reliable, and easy to administer measure of the severity of Achilles tendinopathy and appears to be suitable for both clinical rating and quantitative research.[43] Completion of this questionnaire by the patient can be an additional useful source in information that the clinician can use to make the diagnosis of Achilles tendinopathy.

CLINICAL EXAMINATION

The clinical examination of a patient presenting with symptoms consistent with Achilles tendinopathy should involve both lower extremities. Oftentimes there are subtle changes in the tendon that may not be appreciated unless compared with the contralateral limb. The examination should include muscle strength testing of bilateral superficial posterior muscle groups and an assessment of ankle and subtalar joint range of motion as well as foot position in stance and gait. Equinus due to a gastrocnemius contracture has been associated with the development of Achilles tendinopathy.[44–47] On the contrary, Mahieu and colleagues[48] found that decreased plantarflexion strength and an increased amount of dorsiflexion excursion were significant predictors of Achilles tendon overuse injuries. It is imperative to perform a through clinical examination identifying all biomechanical and musculoskeletal abnormalities because the findings will help to direct treatment recommendations.

Specific findings that have been associated with Achilles tendinopathy include tendon thickening, crepitus, pain on palpation, positive arc sign, and positive Royal London Hospital test. Additionally, there may be difficulty or pain associated with a single-legged heel raise and the hop tests, as well as symptoms with passive stretch of the Achilles.[38,42] When tendon thickening is present, this is most likely a result of the poor reparative process and collagen disarray associated with chronic changes, as noted previously. Crepitus on examination is indicative of paratendinitis, where a fibrous exudate fills the tendon sheath after acute edema and hyperemia of the paratenon with the infiltration of inflammatory cells.[15,49,50]

ARC SIGN

The arc sign is performed by the clinician identifying the intratendinous thickening or swelling of the tendon by palpation and asking the patient to actively dorsiflex and plantarflex the ankle. A positive arc sign is present when the swelling or thickening is visualized to move relative to the malleoli during the active movement.[49] If the thickened portion is not observed to move with active contraction, this is thought to be more indicative of paratendinous (peritendinitis) thickening rather than tendon degeneration.

ROYAL LONDON HOSPITAL TEST

This test is performed with the clinician palpating the tendon to identify an area of local tenderness while the ankle is initially in a neutral or slightly plantarflexed position. The patient is then asked to actively dorsiflex and plantarflex the ankle. A positive finding is when palpation of the tender area of the tendon at rest results in significantly less or no pain at the same location when the ankle is maximally dorsiflexed.[49]

Reiman and colleagues[51] performed a systematic review with meta-analysis of the literature related to the utility of clinical measures for the diagnosis of Achilles tendon injuries. Based on their inclusion criteria, 2 studies were identified that looked at Achilles tendinopathy.[42,49] They found that the subjective measures of pain and morning stiffness, combined with the arc sign, Royal London Hospital test, crepitus, single-legged heel raise, and the presence of tendon thickening when seen together in the same patient could confirm tendinosis of the Achilles. They did caution against using any of these measures independently for diagnosis, as a single finding was unable to consistently confirm the diagnosis.[51] Hutchison and colleagues[42] found high sensitivity (0.780, 0.58–0.94) for self-reported pain, and high sensitivity (0.886, 0.75–0.98) for morning stiffness in their series. Pooled data from the 2 studies found high specificity for palpation (0.81, 0.65–0.91), the arc sign (0.88, 0.74–0.96), and the Royal London Hospital test (0.86, 0.72–0.95), thus the recommendation to combine the subjective and clinical findings to increase the diagnostic ability. They also found the remaining examinations in the examination section to be specific, although not sensitive; however, these were not studied by Maffuli and colleagues.[49]

In their study, Mafulli and colleagues[49] also performed sonographic assessment of the Achilles as a part of the diagnostic workup and all subjects had a histologic diagnosis of Achilles tendinopathy confirmed postoperatively. They concluded in patients with tendinopathy of the Achilles tendon with a tender area of intratendinous swelling that moves with the tendon and whose tenderness significantly decreases or disappears when the tendon is put under tension, a clinical diagnosis of tendinopathy can be formulated, with a high positive predictive chance that the tendon will show ultrasonographic and histologic features of tendinopathy.

In conclusion, tendinopathy consists of several anatomic and histologic findings ranging from paratendinous inflammation to noninflammatory tendon fiber degeneration. Knowledge of the mechanical, structural, and histologic components of this spectrum of disease is vital for proper diagnosis and treatment selection. Clinical examination is the cornerstone of diagnosis with imaging rarely needed, as noted in previous articles. Treatment should be focused on both the structural tendon changes and the potential mechanical causes of inflammation and degeneration.

ACKNOWLEDGMENTS

The author acknowledges the contribution of Matthew Sieloff, BS, College of Podiatric Medicine and Surgery, Des Moines University, in the subject research and assistance writing this article.

REFERENCES

1. Paavola M, Kannus P, Järvinen TAH, et al. Achilles tendinopathy. J Bone Joint Surg Am 2002;84-A(11):2062–76.

2. Maffulli N, Khan KM, Puddu G. Overuse tendon conditions: time to change a confusing terminology. Arthroscopy 1998;14(8):840–3.

3. Khan KM, Cook JL, Taunton JE, et al. Overuse tendinosis, not tendinitis part 1: a new paradigm for a difficult clinical problem. Phys Sportsmed 2000;28(5):38–48.
4. Järvinen TAH, Kannus P, Maffulli N, et al. Achilles tendon disorders: etiology and epidemiology. Foot Ankle Clin 2005;10(2):255–66.
5. Scott A, Khan KM, Duronio V. IGF-I activates PKB and prevents anoxic apoptosis in Achilles tendon cells. J Orthop Res 2005;23(5):1219–25.
6. Maffulli N, Testa V, Capasso G, et al. Similar histopathological picture in males with Achilles and patellar tendinopathy. Med Sci Sports Exerc 2004;36(9):1470–5.
7. Nell E, van der Merwe L, Cook J, et al. The apoptosis pathway and the genetic predisposition to Achilles tendinopathy. J Orthop Res 2012;30(11):1719–24.
8. Alfredson H. The chronic painful Achilles and patellar tendon: research on basic biology and treatment. Scand J Med Sci Sports 2005;15(4):252–9.
9. Alfredson H, Lorentzon R. Chronic Achilles tendinosis: recommendations for treatment and prevention. Sports Med 2000;29(2):135–46.
10. Baker BE. Current concepts in the diagnosis and treatment of musculotendinous injuries. Med Sci Sports Exerc 1984;16(4):323–7.
11. Kannus P, Natri A. Etiology and pathophysiology of tendon ruptures in sports. Scand J Med Sci Sports 1997;7(2):107–12.
12. Kannus P, Józsa L. Histopathological changes preceding spontaneous rupture of a tendon. A controlled study of 891 patients. J Bone Joint Surg Am 1991;73(10): 1507–25.
13. Józsa L, Kvist M, Bálint BJ, et al. The role of recreational sport activity in Achilles tendon rupture. A clinical, pathoanatomical, and sociological study of 292 cases. Am J Sports Med 1989;17(3):338–43.
14. Tallon C, Maffulli N, Ewen SW. Ruptured Achilles tendons are significantly more degenerated than tendinopathic tendons. Med Sci Sports Exerc 2001;33(12): 1983–90.
15. Maffulli N, Wong J, Almekinders LC. Types and epidemiology of tendinopathy. Clin Sports Med 2003;22(4):675–92.
16. September AV, Nell E, O'Connell K, et al. A pathway-based approach investigating the genes encoding interleukin-1β, interleukin-6 and the interleukin-1 receptor antagonist provides new insight into the genetic susceptibility of Achilles tendinopathy. Br J Sports Med 2011;45(13):1040–7.
17. Holmes GB, Lin J. Etiologic factors associated with symptomatic Achilles tendinopathy. Foot Ankle Int 2006;27(11):952–9.
18. Corrao G, Zambon A, Bertù L, et al. Evidence of tendinitis provoked by fluoroquinolone treatment: a case-control study. Drug Saf 2006;29(10):889–96.
19. van der Linden PD, van de Lei J, Nab HW, et al. Achilles tendinitis associated with fluoroquinolones. Br J Clin Pharmacol 1999;48(3):433–7.
20. Vora AM, Myerson MS, Oliva F, et al. Tendinopathy of the main body of the Achilles tendon. Foot Ankle Clin 2005;10(2):293–308.
21. Williams DS, Zambardino JA, Banning VA. Transverse-plane mechanics at the knee and tibia in runners with and without a history of Achilles tendonopathy. J Orthop Sports Phys Ther 2008;38(12):761–7.
22. Roche AJ, Calder JD. Achilles tendinopathy: a review of the current concepts of treatment. Bone Joint J 2013;95-B(10):1299–307.
23. Courville XF, Coe MP, Hecht PJ. Current concepts review: noninsertional Achilles tendinopathy. Foot Ankle Int 2009;30(11):1132–42.
24. Yang X, Coleman DP, Pugh ND, et al. The volume of the neovascularity and its clinical implications in Achilles tendinopathy. Ultrasound Med Biol 2012;38(11): 1887–95.

25. de Vos R, Weir A, Cobben LPJ, et al. The value of power Doppler ultrasonography in Achilles tendinopathy: a prospective study. Am J Sports Med 2007;35(10): 1696–701.
26. Aström M, Westlin N. Blood flow in chronic Achilles tendinopathy. Clin Orthop Relat Res 1994;(308):166–72.
27. Aström M, Westlin N. No effect of piroxicam on Achilles tendinopathy. A randomized study of 70 patients. Acta Orthop Scand 1992;63(6):631–4.
28. Ohberg L, Alfredson H. Ultrasound guided sclerosis of neovessels in painful chronic Achilles tendinosis: pilot study of a new treatment. Br J Sports Med 2002;36(3):177.
29. Richards PJ, McCall IW, Day C, et al. Longitudinal microvascularity in Achilles tendinopathy (power Doppler ultrasound, magnetic resonance imaging time-intensity curves and the Victorian Institute of Sport Assessment-Achilles Questionnaire): a pilot study. Skeletal Radiol 2010;39(6):509–21.
30. Knobloch K. The role of tendon microcirculation in Achilles and patellar tendinopathy. J Orthop Surg Res 2008;3:18.
31. Alfredson H, Thorsen K, Lorentzon R. In situ microdialysis in tendon tissue: high levels of glutamate, but not prostaglandin E2 in chronic Achilles tendon pain. Knee Surg Sports Traumatol Arthrosc 1999;7(6):378–81.
32. Scott A, Alfredson H, Forsgren S. VGluT2 expression in painful Achilles and patellar tendinosis: evidence of local glutamate release by tenocytes. J Orthop Res 2008;26(5):685–92.
33. Bjur D, Alfredson H, Forsgren S. Presence of the neuropeptide Y1 receptor in tenocytes and blood vessel walls in the human Achilles tendon. Br J Sports Med 2009;43(14):1136–42.
34. Alfredson H, Bjur D, Thorsen K, et al. High intratendinous lactate levels in painful chronic Achilles tendinosis. An investigation using microdialysis technique. J Orthop Res 2002;20(5):934–8.
35. Bjur D, Danielson P, Alfredson H, et al. Presence of a non-neuronal cholinergic system and occurrence of up- and down-regulation in expression of M2 muscarinic acetylcholine receptors: new aspects of importance regarding Achilles tendon tendinosis (tendinopathy). Cell Tissue Res 2008;331(2):385–400.
36. Andersson G, Danielson P, Alfredson H, et al. Nerve-related characteristics of ventral paratendinous tissue in chronic Achilles tendinosis. Knee Surg Sports Traumatol Arthrosc 2007;15(10):1272–9.
37. Schubert TE, Weidler C, Lerch K, et al. Achilles tendinosis is associated with sprouting of substance P positive nerve fibres. Ann Rheum Dis 2005;64(7): 1083–6.
38. Carcia CR, Martin RL, Houck J, et al. Achilles pain, stiffness, and muscle power deficits: Achilles tendinitis. J Orthop Sports Phys Ther 2010;40(9):1.
39. Benjamin M, Toumi H, Ralphs JR, et al. Where tendons and ligaments meet bone: attachment sites ('entheses') in relation to exercise and/or mechanical load. J Anat 2006;208(4):471–90.
40. Brewer BJ. Athletic injuries; musculotendinous unit. Clin Orthop 1962;23:30–8.
41. Cazeau C, Stiglitz Y. Effects of gastrocnemius tightness on forefoot during gait. Foot Ankle Clin 2014;19(4):649–57.
42. Hutchison A, Evans R, Bodger O, et al. What is the best clinical test for Achilles tendinopathy? Foot Ankle Surg 2013;19(2):112–7.
43. Robinson JM, Cook JL, Purdam C, et al. The VISA-A questionnaire: a valid and reliable index of the clinical severity of Achilles tendinopathy. Br J Sports Med 2001;35(5):335–41.

44. Gurdezi S, Kohls-Gatzoulis J, Solan MC. Results of proximal medial gastrocnemius release for Achilles tendinopathy. Foot Ankle Int 2013;34(10):1364–9.
45. Kiewiet NJ, Holthusen SM, Bohay DR, et al. Gastrocnemius recession for chronic noninsertional Achilles tendinopathy. Foot Ankle Int 2013;34(4):481–5.
46. Laborde JM, Weiler L. Achilles tendon pain treated with gastrocnemius-soleus recession. Orthopedics 2011;34(4):289–91.
47. Kaufman KR, Brodine SK, Shaffer RA, et al. The effect of foot structure and range of motion on musculoskeletal overuse injuries. Am J Sports Med 1999;27(5): 585–93.
48. Mahieu NN, Witvrouw E, Stevens V, et al. Intrinsic risk factors for the development of Achilles tendon overuse injury: a prospective study. Am J Sports Med 2006; 34(2):226–35.
49. Maffulli N, Kenward M, Testa V, et al. Clinical diagnosis of Achilles tendinopathy with tendinosis. Clin J Sport Med 2003;13(1):11–5.
50. Kvist M, Józsa L, Järvinen M, et al. Fine structural alterations in chronic Achilles paratenonitis in athletes. Pathol Res Pract 1985;180(4):416–23.
51. Reiman M, Burgi C, Strube E, et al. The utility of clinical measures for the diagnosis of Achilles tendon injuries: a systematic review with meta-analysis. J Athl Train 2014;49(6):820–9.

Nonsurgical Management of Midsubstance Achilles Tendinopathy

 CrossMark

Shane McClinton, DPT, OCS, CSCS[a],*,
Lace Luedke, DPT, PhD, OCS, CSCS[b], Derek Clewley, DPT, OCS[c]

KEYWORDS

- Tendinosis • Tendonitis • Eccentric • Posterior heel pain • Midportion

KEY POINTS

- Achilles tendinopathy is commonly due to a change in activity level, but may also be related to pathoanatomic, biomechanical, and pain-related impairments.
- Reactive tendon states require acute symptom management strategies in contrast to treatment for a tendon in disrepair or degeneration.
- Tendon loading exercise is the mainstay of initial management, but may be supported by medication, ice, shoe inserts, manual therapy, stretching, taping, or low-level laser.
- If unresponsive to initial management, shockwave therapy and injections are options before considering surgery.
- The Victorian Institute of Sports Assessment-Achilles, pain scales, heel raise and jump tests, and ultrasound can be used to assess treatment outcome and recovery.

INTRODUCTION

The Achilles tendon is one of the most commonly injured tendons that results in significant pain and loss of function. The incidence of Achilles tendinopathy (AT) is 2.35 per 1000 in the adult population and is frequently associated with sporting activities or a change in activity level.[1] Men and women between the ages of 20 and 60 are affected equally and commonly present to a health care provider 11 to 12 weeks after the onset of symptoms.[1] A variety of etiologic factors contribute to AT and a thorough

Disclosure Statement: The authors have nothing to disclose.
[a] Doctor of Physical Therapy Program, Des Moines University, 3200 Grand Avenue, Des Moines, IA 50312, USA; [b] Kinesiology Department, University of Wisconsin-Oshkosh, 108B Albee Hall, 800 Algoma Boulevard, Oshkosh, WI 54901, USA; [c] Division of Doctor of Physical Therapy, Duke University, 2200 West Main Street, B-230, Durham, NC 27705, USA
* Corresponding author.
E-mail address: shane.mcclinton@dmu.edu

Clin Podiatr Med Surg 34 (2017) 137–160
http://dx.doi.org/10.1016/j.cpm.2016.10.004
0891-8422/17/© 2016 Elsevier Inc. All rights reserved.

evaluation combined with evidence of treatment effectiveness and the patient's preferences are important to identify the most appropriate treatment plan. Treatment is often successful with nonsurgical intervention, and some unresponsive cases may be candidates for surgery.[2] The purpose of this article is to describe the nonsurgical management of midsubstance AT.

PATIENT EVALUATION OVERVIEW

The etiology of midsubstance AT is variable and often multifactorial. Evidence-informed evaluation will help to identify relevant factors in each patient with AT and devise appropriate treatment. Etiologic factors include overuse, training errors, altered lower limb biomechanics, footwear, postural or leg length imbalances, impaired muscle performance, and direct trauma.[2–6] In addition to etiologic factors, the status of the tendon is important in treatment decisions and prognosis. The continuum model of tendinopathy provides a simple way of estimating tendon status and can be used in parallel with examination findings and treatment (**Fig. 1**).[7] Of particular importance is dissociating tendon reactivity from disrepair or degeneration. Clinically, a reactive tendon is acutely painful even to minimal load, has homogenous swelling (no lumps or bumps), and the patient reports a substantial change in activity that overloaded the tendon. Other considerations important to diagnosis, treatment, and prognosis include biomechanical, pathoanatomic, and pain characteristics identified using clinical measures and imaging (**Table 1**).

History and Comorbidities

- Frequently associated with sporting activities, but can occur in nonathletes.
- Tendon reaction induced by change in activity level, including increased training volume, intensity, or terrain (eg, hill training). Reactivity may be induced after a period of immobilization (eg, recovering from injury), decreased activity (eg, off-season), initiating an exercise program from a relatively sedentary lifestyle, or a direct trauma to the Achilles.[3,6]
- Individuals with diabetes, obesity, dyslipidemia, inflammatory or autoimmune disorders, hypertension, and prior use of oral or injected steroids are at increased risk.[1,24–26]

State of the Achilles Tendon

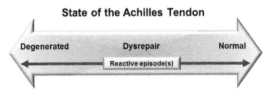

Fig. 1. Continuum model of load-induced tendinopathy.[7] Clinically, a reactive tendon results in pain and acute reaction in the tendon cell and extracellular matrix after a burst of unaccustomed physical activity (including after immobilization) or a direct blow. Reactivity can present on a previously normal tendon or on a tendon in disrepair or degenerated. In tendon disrepair, failed or incomplete attempts to heal from the reactive stage results in further, but reversible, changes in the tendon matrix with or without vascular and neural ingrowth. The degenerative tendon demonstrates additional cellular and matrix changes (see pathoanatomic characteristics in **Table 1**) some of which are irreversible. Treatment for Achilles tendinopathy attempts to manage reactive episodes with a long-term goal of shifting the tendon state toward normal.

Table 1
Characteristics that have been described in individuals with Achilles tendinopathy and associated method of measurement

Characteristics of Individuals with AT	Method of Measurement
Pathoanatomic	
Increased tendon echogenicity heterogeneity[8,9]	Ultrasound
Increased tendon CSA and thickness[9,10]	Ultrasound and MRI
Tendon softening[11]	Ultrasound elastography
Partial tearing[9]	Ultrasound and MRI
Neovascularization[12]	Doppler ultrasound
Biomechanical	
Decreased (<11.5°)[13] or increased (>9°)[14] ankle dorsiflexion measured with knee extended	Goniometer
Increased rearfoot inversion measured in non–weight-bearing,[13] and at initial contact of running[15]	Goniometer and 3D motion analysis
Increased rearfoot eversion,[15,16] inversion–eversion total range of motion[16] and rate of eversion[15] during running	3D motion analysis
Subtalar varus ≥4° or forefoot varus of ≥3° measured in non–weight-bearing[17]	Goniometer
Decreased ankle plantar flexion strength[14,15,18]	Isokinetic dynomometer
Decreased ankle plantar flexion power[19]	Spring loaded string/linear encoder
Decreased jump height and increased jump contact time[19]	Force mat
Decreased tendon stiffness[20]	Dynamic ultrasound and isometric dynamometer
Increased tendon strain[21]	Dynamic ultrasound and isometric dynamometer
Pain-related mechanisms	
Decreased tactile acuity[22]	2-point discrimination using asthesiometer
Increased local and nonlocal mechanical hyperalgesia[23]	Pain-pressure threshold using algometer

Abbreviations: 3D, 3-dimensional; AT, Achilles tendinopathy; CSA, cross-sectional area.

Palpation

- Palpatory tenderness is a hallmark sign of AT. The tendon is palpated by squeezing the Achilles tendon between the thumb and index finger with the patient prone.
- Pain and tenderness 2 to 6 cm from the distal attachment (Sp 0.73, +LR 3.11) that decreases with palpation in maximum dorsiflexion (aka, Royal London test; Sp 0.93, +LR 7.29)[27] helps to confirm the diagnosis.

- In chronic tendinopathy, there is a region of tendon thickening (Sp 0.90, +LR 5.90).[27]
- Swelling that moves distally during dorsiflexion and proximally during plantar flexion may be observed (aka, arc sign; Sp 1.0, +LR infinity).[27]
- Pain increases with activity and stiffness is reported during initial steps after being at rest.[3] Increased stiffness perceived by patient is different from biomechanical stiffness, which is reduced in tendinopathy.[20]
- Lack of pain with palpation (Sn 0.84, -LR 0.22) and no morning stiffness (Sn 0.89, -LR 0.19) are the 2 best single-item tests to rule out AT.

Ankle Plantar Flexor Muscle Performance

- Ankle plantar flexor muscle performance may be impaired owing to altered tendon structure or compensatory movement.
- Limited plantar flexion strength and power has been associated with AT using isokinetic dynamometery,[14,15,18,19] but repeated single leg heel raises are the simplest method to assess plantar flexor muscle performance in the clinic.
- Standardized heel raise height by touching the dorsum of the foot to a crossbar (see **Fig. 3**F) improves the ability to identify plantar flexor impairments, including side-to-side differences.[19]
- Athletes less than 40 years of age perform 20 to 25 single-leg heel raises on average,[19] but fewer repetitions are expected for nonathletes and older individuals.[28]
- Pain during single leg heel raise testing is specific for AT (SP 0.93, +LR 3.14).[27]

Ankle and Foot Posture and Mobility

- There is conflicting evidence of ankle dorsiflexion impairments (see **Table 1**),[13,14] and therefore side-to-side differences may be more important in decision making. In the late stages of disrepair or degeneration, there may be increased dorsiflexion owing to increased tendon compliance. Dorsiflexion can be measured reliably in the supine or prone position with the foot off the plinth and the knee extended and then flexed at least 45°.[29]
- Static foot posture can be assessed and compared with the uninvolved side using the foot posture or arch height indices.[30–32] Although tendinopathy may be present with any foot type, the Achilles may be susceptible to injury with increased foot pronation owing to its orientation medial to the subtalar joint axis and decreased tolerance to frontal and transverse plane motion.[33]
- Impaired mobility of the rearfoot (inversion or eversion) and ankle (dorsiflexion) may alter tendon loading during activity and has been identified primarily in runners and military trainees (see **Table 1**).[13–16]
- Video analysis may help to identify rearfoot and ankle movement impairments (eg, eversion and toe-out angle). A standardized analysis includes the use of a treadmill for gait analysis, capture rate of at least 120 frames/s for running or jumping (30 frames/s for walking), and camera placed perpendicular to the patient from posterior and lateral perspectives. During jumping, special attention is paid to side-to-side differences in heel height.
- Foot posture and mobility may be affected by function of proximal regions and considered in the evaluation. Dynamic knee and rearfoot valgus may be owing to altered neuromotor function of the gluteal muscles (ie, hip abductors and external rotators) and can be assessed by performance of single leg squat/step down or manual muscle tests.[4,5,34]

Imaging

- Tendon heterogeneity, thickening, softening, tearing, and neovascularization have been identified using ultrasound imaging or MRI and may help to indicate the degree of tendon disrepair or degeneration (see **Table 1**).[8–12]
- Although imaging results may indicate the degree of pathoanatomic changes, this does not always correlate with symptom severity or improvement.[35] Therefore, careful use of imaging and discussion of results are important to avoid negative impacts on fear–avoidance behaviors and treatment expectations.

PHARMACOLOGIC TREATMENT OPTIONS

Pharmacologic treatment including oral, topical, and injected interventions can modulate symptoms and tissue healing to manage reactive tendon states (see **Fig. 1**) and complement a tendon loading program in nonacute tendinopathy (**Fig. 2**). Various pharmacologic treatments have been used in AT and no pharmacologic treatment, when used in isolation, has proven superior to a tendon loading exercise program.[36] With the exception of an acute, reactive tendinopathy in an otherwise healthy tendon, pharmacologic treatment of AT is more effective when combined with a tendon loading exercise program.[36] Fluoroquinolone antibiotics, oral corticosteroids, low-molecular-weight heparin, and the use of cyclosporine, cortisone, and rapamycin after organ transplant have been linked to AT and should be considered when taking the patient history or used with caution if indicated.[37–40]

Nonsteroidal Antiinflammatory Drugs: Oral and Topical

- Although AT generally lacks inflammatory cells, NSAIDs have both antiinflammatory and analgesic effects and may be used in acute or reactive tendon states.[42] Laboratory studies indicate that NSAIDs may improve tensile strength of tendons via increasing cross-linkages between collagen fibers but the effect of NSAIDS on fibroblasts could potentially cause inflammatory and degenerative changes.[43]
- Oral NSAIDs are not recommended for chronic tendinopathy,[44–46] but may be effective for short-term (7–14 days) pain relief[44,45]
- Numerous NSAID options are available (**Table 2**), and none have superior effectiveness for AT. Although ibuprofen has a lesser risk of gastrointestinal side effects, naproxen or celecoxib may be preferred for those with cardiovascular risk factors.[53]
- The side effects of NSAIDs include gastrointestinal and cardiovascular distress and should be used as briefly as possible.[45,46,53]
- Topical NSAIDs, such as diclofenac gel, are an effective and safe alternative to oral NSAIDs to reduce pain associated with acute tendinopathy.[54,55]

Injections

- Injected agents can modulate symptoms and/or facilitate tissue healing, but there is insufficient evidence to support routine use as the sole intervention.[49]
- Recent systematic reviews have concluded that platelet-rich plasma is not supported for AT[56,57]
- Local injection of corticosteroids may be useful in acute reactive AT to reduce pain and enable tendon loading exercise,[41] but has little evidence for benefit in midsubstance AT and increases risk of rupture, especially in degenerated tendons.[45,58,59]
- Injected vascular sclerosing agents are used in chronic tendinopathy to address neovascularization and corresponding nerves to reduce pain.[41,60] Because of

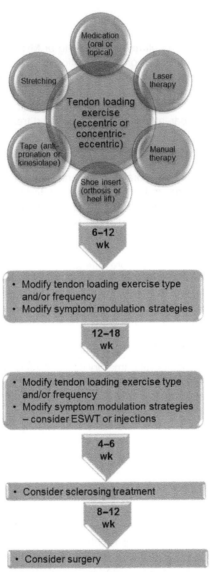

Fig. 2. Treatment pathway for the management of midportion Achilles tendinopathy adapted from recommendations by Alfredson and Cook.[41] Timeframes and intervention may be adjusted to consider the patient's preferences, presentation, and response to initial treatment. If patient responds satisfactorily to any phase of treatment, loading exercises should be maintained for 6 to 12 months and symptom modulation strategies as needed. ESWT, extracorporeal shock wave therapy.

conflicting evidence of effectiveness,[60–63] the need for several injections, and procedures that are technically demanding, sclerosing agents are considered after unsuccessful treatment with a tendon loading exercise program (see **Fig 2**).[41,64]

- When warranted, specific procedures for injection intervention in the management of AT are described by Smith and colleagues. (See W. Bret Smith and colleagues' article, "Midsubstance Tendinopathy, Percutaneous Techniques

Table 2
Pharmacologic treatment options

Medication	Application	Usual Dosing	Frequency	Duration
Nitrates				
Glyceryl trinitrate[38,47,48]	Topical patch	1.25 mg[a]/24 h	Replace patch daily	12–24 wk
Sclerosing agent				
Polidocanol[49]	Ultrasound + Doppler-guided injections	5–10 mg/mL	1–5 injections	3–6 wk apart
Steroids				
Dexamethasone[50]	Iontophoresis	3 mL 80 mA-min	4 treatments	Every 3–4 d over 2 wk
Triamcinalone[49,51]	Ultrasound-guided peritendinous injection	20 mg with 3.5 mL of 1% lidocaine or 3.5 mL 0.5% bupivicaine	1 time	–
Methylprednisolone[52]	Peritendinous Injection	40 mg in 1 mL of 0.25% marcaine	1 time	–
NSAIDs				
Aspirin[53]	Oral	325–650 mg	QID	7–14 d[45]
Diclofenac[53]	Oral	50–75 mg	BID	7–14 d[45]
Etodolac[53]	Oral	200–400 mg	TID–QID	7–14 d[45]
Ibuprofen[53]	Oral	200–800 mg	TID–QID	7–14 d[45]
Indomethacin[53]	Oral	20–50 mg	TID	7–14 d[45]
Meloxicam[53]	Oral	7.5–15 mg	Daily	7–14 d[45]
Nabumetone[53]	Oral	1000 mg	Daily	7–14 d[45]
Naproxen[53]	Oral	250–500 mg	BID	7–14 d[45]
Piroxicam[53]	Oral	20 mg/d	Daily	7–14 d[45]
Sulindac[53]	Oral	150–200 mg	BID	7–14 d[45]
Celecoxib[53]	Oral	100–200 mg	BID	7–14 d[45]
Diclofenac sodium 1% gel[54]	Topical	2–4 g	QID, Maximum of 32 g/d over affected areas	7–14 d

Abbreviations: BID, twice daily; NSAIDs, nonsteroidal antiinflmmatory drugs; QID, 4 times a day; TID, 3 times a day.
[a] A 5-mg patch cut into fourths.

(Platelet-Rich Plasma, Extracorporeal Shock Wave Therapy, Prolotherapy, Radiofrequency Ablation)," in this issue.)

Topical Agents

- Agents administered topically such as glyceryl trinitrate patch and iontophoresis with dexamethasone may be effective in acute or reactive tendinopathy, but have not been studied as isolated interventions.
- Topical agents are coupled with a tendon loading exercise program, especially in reactive tendon states with suspected dysrepair or degeneration.

NONPHARMACOLOGIC TREATMENT OPTIONS

The most extensively studied and effective nonpharmacologic treatment for midsubstance AT is tendon loading exercise. Several other interventions have been investigated when combined with a tendon loading program, but few have been studied in isolation and none have demonstrated superior effects to a tendon loading program. Therefore, tendon loading exercises such as eccentric and concentric–eccentric heel raises form the core of midsubstance AT management (see **Fig. 2**) and the majority of patients can have a successful long-term outcome.[65] Several different training programs have been proposed that vary in the type and speed of exercise in addition to the dosage and magnitude of loading (**Table 3**). There is limited evidence directly comparing the different tendon loading programs and no program has proven superior to the others. Therefore, consideration of the literature and patient preferences can help to identify the most appropriate loading program that the patient will adhere to for the time necessary to complete the program. To manage symptoms and facilitate adherence to the tendon loading program, there are several symptom-modulating interventions (see **Fig. 2**) discussed in the Combination Therapies Section that can be used, depending on patient preference and response. In addition, etiologic factors identified from the history and examination is important to address in the overall treatment plan. A physical therapist may assist in identifying the most appropriate tendon loading program, appropriate progression of loading, etiologic factors to address, and implementing symptom and physiologic modulating interventions if needed.

Correction of Etiologic Factors

- In acute reactive states in an otherwise healthy tendon, rest from activity that originally overloaded the tendon or reduced tendon load is warranted. The most common training factors in midsubstance AT include a rapid increase in activity/training such as initiating or progressing an exercise program, introducing sprint/interval training, or adding hill training.
- Other biomechanical factors associated with midsubstance AT are listed in **Table 1**. With the exception of trauma, most biomechanical factors arise gradually and are addressed with combined intervention, including taping, foot orthoses, and specific exercise interventions.

Tendon Loading Exercise

- The most common tendon loading exercises for the Achilles include heel raises using eccentric and concentric–eccentric muscle contractions (**Fig. 3**). Loading exercises are progressed by increasing load and speed depending on recreational and functional demands.
- Isolated eccentric exercises have been used in multiple clinical trials and significantly improved pain and function,[66] although evidence is limited that eccentrics are superior to other loading programs.[73,74] Other loading programs include

Table 3
Parameters of tendon loading programs using heel raises (see Fig. 3)

Tendon Loading Program	Exercise Description	Load/Progression	Sets × Repetitions	Frequency
Isolated eccentric[18,66] First week transition variation[67,68] Do as tolerated variation[69]	Standing with heels off the edge of a step, raise heels up using both feet (see Fig. 3C) and slowly[a] lower using only 1 leg (see Fig 3D). Perform with knees straight and flexed approximately 45°.	Body weight at first, add weight using a backpack or by holding dumbbells when exercise becomes pain free (stop if disabling)	Knee straight: 3 × 15 Knee flexed: 3 × 15 Week 1: Knee straight only. Day 1–2: 1 × 10–15, day 3–4: 2 × 15, day 5–7: 3 × 15. Weeks 2–12: 3 × 15 with knee straight and 3 × 15 with knee flexed Goal of 3 × 15 with knee straight and 3 × 15 with knee bent, but patient can perform a repetition volume that is tolerable	2 times/d, 7 d/wk for 12 wk

(continued on next page)

Table 3
(continued)

Tendon Loading Program	Exercise Description	Load/Progression	Sets × Repetitions	Frequency
Combined eccentric, concentric, and plyometric[3,70,71]	Standing heel raises Standing with heels on floor or off the edge of a step, raise heel(s) up and slowly[a] lower. For eccentric heel raises, raise up with both feet and slowly[a] lower using only 1 leg. Seated heel raises In the seated position raise 1 heel up and slowly[a] lower. Quick rebounding heel raises Standing with heels on floor, raise and lower heels quickly as if you are jumping without the toes leaving the floor. Turn back up when the heel is approximately 1 cm from the floor.	Body weight at first, add weight using a backpack, weight machine, or by holding dumbbells. Adjust load or do not advance to the step if more than 5/10 pain during, or in the 24 hours after exercise	Weeks 1–2 (Phase 1): Two- and then one-legged heel raises from floor, seated heel raises, and eccentric heel raises from floor: 3 × 10 each Weeks 2–5 (Phase 2): Same as Phase I, but all heel raises performed on edge of step: 3 × 15 each; and add quick rebounding heel raises from floor: 3 × 20 Weeks 3–12 (Phase 3): Same as Phase II but add weight (except during quick rebounding heel raises); and add plyometrics Weeks 12–26 (Phase 4): Continue one-legged and eccentric heel raises on step with weight: 3 × 15; and quick rebounding heel raises 3 × 20	Phase 1: 1 time/d Phase 2: 1 time/d Phase 3: 2–3 times/wk Phase 4: 2–3 times/wk

| Heavy slow resistance[72] | Heel raises performed with a 3-s concentric and 3-s eccentric phase (6 s total): (1) on a seated calf raise machine with knees flexed 90°, (2) on a leg press machine with knees straight, and (3) standing with heels off of a 1.5-inch object, barbell on shoulders and knees straight. | Progressed based on 15, 12, 10, 8, and 6 RM in respective training weeks. Pain rated at 4–5/10 allowable during training if subsided before the next session. | 3–4 sets with a 2–3 min rest between sets and 5 min rest between exercise. Week 1: 3 × 15 RM, Weeks 2–3: 3 × 12 RM, Weeks 4–5: 4 × 10 RM, Weeks 6–8: 4 × 8 RM, Weeks 9–12: 4 × 6 RM | 3 times/wk for 12 wk |

Abbreviation: RM, repetition maximum.

[a] Speed is not described in most studies, but 3 seconds per repetition has been suggested.[72]

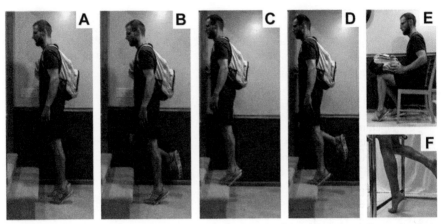

Fig. 3. Heel raise exercise performed (*A*) bilaterally on the floor, (*B*) unilaterally on the floor, (*C*) bilaterally on a step, (*D*) unilaterally on a step, and (*E*) seated. Isolated eccentric exercise is performed by performing the concentric phase bilaterally (*A* or *C*) and the eccentric phase unilaterally (*B* or *E*). Weight can be added to a backpack to increase load. Standardization of heel raise height during testing is achieved by the dorsum of the foot touching a bar at the peak of each repetition (*F*).

heavy slow resistance training, a do-as-tolerated eccentric loading, and a combined program including isolated eccentrics, concentric–eccentric, and plyometric exercise (see **Table 3**).

- If evidence of hip (contralateral pelvic drop, dynamic knee valgus) or foot weakness (pronation) is observed, specific exercise advised by a physical therapist may be warranted. Impaired gluteal muscle performance has been identified in runners with AT and may be related to the cause or persistence of symptoms.[4,5]
- Education about expected pain responses and recovery time is essential to the tendon loading program. Increased fear of movement may have a negative effect on exercise effectiveness,[65] although this can be mitigated through appropriate education. Patients should be informed that muscle soreness is expected during the first few weeks,[18] although the program can be adapted by reduced volume and a gradual transition in the first week.[67,68]
- Pain in the tendon is normal and an expected part of the loading program. A pain monitoring model can be used to guide intensity of training.[3,70] In this model, pain of less than 5 on a scale of 0 (no pain) to 10 (worst imaginable pain) is acceptable during or within the 24 hours after training. If pain is greater than 5 out of 10 or pain and perceived stiffness is progressing from 1 week to the next, then the magnitude, volume, or dosage of loading should be modified.
- Soreness may be mitigated through use of symptom modulating interventions, such as medication, manual therapy, ice, stretching, taping, or shoe inserts.

Shoe Inserts

- Foot orthoses may be effective to alter the biomechanical and pain-related characteristics, but evidence is limited to runners.[75,76] Although foot orthoses are intended typically to reduce pain through control of pronation, actual kinematic changes may not be necessary to achieve symptomatic improvement.[76] Neuromotor changes in the foot and calf muscles associated with foot orthoses use may also contribute to symptomatic improvement.[77]

- There is conflicting evidence on the use of heel lifts,[33] but recent evidence indicates that heel lifts may decrease compressive strain associated with AT and may be helpful during a reactive episode.[78]

COMBINATION THERAPIES

Tendon loading exercise is the foundation of nonsurgical treatment for midsubstance AT, but can be combined with other symptom and physiologic modifying interventions to facilitate recovery (see **Fig. 2**).[3] Several pharmacologic and nonpharmacologic interventions have been used with varying degrees of effectiveness to produce short-term changes in pain, perceived stiffness, and healing. Choosing between the various interventions to couple with tendon loading exercise should consider the clinical presentation that estimates the state of the tendon (see **Fig. 1**), including reactivity, availability of equipment, the patient's preferences, and prior response to treatment.

Tendon Loading Exercise and Laser Therapy

The addition of low-level laser therapy to an isolated eccentric tendon loading program has demonstrated conflicting results, in part, owing to varying methodology.[79,80] Parameters for laser therapy include irradiation of 6 points 1 cm apart on each side of the painful tendon with 0.91 J/point using an 820 nm wavelength probe that results in a power density of 60 mW/cm^2 for 12 total sessions over 6 weeks.[79] The use of low-level laser therapy may be restricted owing to limited access to laser devices in most clinics.[2] If used, effectiveness may be reduced if the patient has previously been treated with a steroid injection or if higher power densities greater than 100 mW/cm^2 are used.[79]

Tendon Loading Exercise and Iontophoresis

In individuals with less than 3 months of pain, evidence from 1 small study indicates that dexamethasone delivered via iontophoresis may improve pain at 6 months and 1 year when coupled with a concentric-eccentric tendon loading and stretching program.[50] A dose of 80 mA•min (20 minutes at 4 mA if tolerated) can be delivered using 3 mL of dexamethasone 4 times during a 2-week period.[50]

Tendon Loading Exercise and Shoe Inserts

No studies were found that analyzed foot orthoses or heel lifts in addition to tendon loading exercises, but they may be beneficial for short-term use in the patient who has biomechanical deficits or who demonstrates improvement in pain with a trial of foot orthoses or a heel lift.[75-78] Particularly, a heel lift may be effective if the tendon is reactive, but should be weaned as the tendon state improves (see **Fig. 1**). In addition, antipronation taping may be an effective strategy to predict symptomatic response to the use of foot orthoses.[81,82]

Tendon Loading Exercise and Taping

In addition to the use of antipronation tape, there is limited and conflicting evidence that kinesiology tape can reduce symptoms in individuals with midsubstance AT.[83,84] Considering the low cost and low risk of this intervention, kinesiology tape may be used to modulate symptoms when used in conjunction with a tendon loading program. Tape is applied parallel to the Achilles from the posterior calcaneus to the proximal lower leg using 1 or 2 strips. Tape can be left on for a few hours up to 1 week depending on patient tolerance and initial treatment response.[84,85]

Tendon Loading Exercise and Manual therapy

Manual therapy based on joint and soft tissue impairments may help to improve function and adherence to tendon loading exercises by managing the musculotendon soreness associated with repeated tendon loading.[33] Soft tissue mobilization is commonly performed parallel to the calf musculotendon fiber direction with or without a mobilization tool, or perpendicular to the tendon during dorsiflexion and plantar flexion.[33,86–88] When indicated, direct mobilization of the tendon should be performed with caution to avoid a reactive response and should not be performed if the tendon is in a reactive state. Specific attention to tender and taut bands (trigger points) in the calf muscles can help to address sources of referred pain to the Achilles tendon.[88,89] Trigger or tender points can be treated in a variety of ways including ischemic pressure, transverse friction, longitudinal strokes along the trigger band with 1 end "pinned," or trigger point dry needling, depending on clinician experience and the patient's preference. In addition to the calf, impairments in the posterior thigh, quadriceps, and gluteal area may be considered in select cases if associated with the AT.[4,5,88]

Tendon Loading Exercise and Stretching

Calf stretches may help to reduce soreness and calf tightness associated with midsubstance AT, especially in individuals with limited dorsiflexion.[33] Stretches are performed with the knee straight and with the knee bent for 30-second holds.[90]

Tendon Loading Exercise and Cryotherapy

Cold or ice packs applied before and/or after activity, including tendon loading exercises, can help to reduce symptoms, particularly when the tendon is in a reactive state.[75,91]

Tendon Loading Exercise and Topical Glyceryl Trinitrate

Topical glyceryl trinitrate (TGTN) is purported to promote tendon healing via the influence of nitric oxide on blood flow, collagen synthesis, and cellular adhesion, in addition to its analgesic effects.[45,47,53] Studies demonstrate conflicting results when TGTN is combined with an eccentric loading program in individuals with chronic AT, with some reporting improved symptoms and function and another showing no benefit.[47,48,92] Studies included application of a TGTN patch every 24 hours for 6 months to the most painful area. The effectiveness of intermittent use of the TGTN patch is unknown and side effects include skin rash at the patch site and headache, which may limit adherence to treatment.[2]

Tendon Loading Exercise and Shockwave Therapy

Low-energy shockwave therapy can provide additional benefit when added to eccentric exercises.[67,93] If the equipment is available, shockwave therapy may be considered if the patient is slow to respond to tendon loading exercise.[94] Specific procedures for Shockwave therapy are described by Smith and colleagues. (See W. Bret Smith and colleagues' article, "Midsubstance Tendinopathy, Percutaneous Techniques (Platelet-Rich Plasma, Extracorporeal Shock Wave Therapy, Prolotherapy, Radiofrequency Ablation)," in this issue.)

Tendon Loading Exercise and Injections

Despite limited evidence to support injection therapy for midsubstance AT,[49] injections may be worthwhile when coupled with tendon loading exercises. Commonly used agents include corticosteroids, hypertonic glucose (prolotherapy), platelet-rich plasma, and polidocanol (a sclerosing agent).[49] Because of limited evidence of effectiveness over nonpharmacologic treatment, injections are reserved for cases not responsive to initial management. Specific procedures for injection therapies are described by Smith and colleagues. (See W. Bret Smith and colleagues' article, "Midsubstance Tendinopathy, Percutaneous Techniques (Platelet-Rich Plasma, Extracorporeal Shock Wave Therapy, Prolotherapy, Radiofrequency Ablation)," in this issue.)

Tendon Loading Exercise and Bracing

Daily use of the DonJoy AirHeel brace (DonJoy Performance, Vista, CA) did not provide any additional benefit to eccentric exercises.[95] Bracing may be considered in a very reactive tendon state where walking is affected severely. The duration of bracing should be limited to avoid decline in strength and stiffness properties of the tendon,[96,97] and early loading after bracing used to promote tendon remodeling.[98]

Tendon Loading Exercise and Night Splints

Night splints provide inferior improvements in pain and function when compared with an eccentric tendon loading program and do not provide any additional benefit when added to an eccentric program.[68,99,100]

TREATMENT RESISTANCE AND COMPLICATIONS

The majority of patients will recover with treatment that includes tendon loading exercise, but 10% to 30% will continue to have symptoms.[65,101] Resistance to treatment may be owing to nonadherence to treatment recommendations, severity of tendon degeneration, or sensitization. Although tendon properties change with age, patients of older age, and longer duration or higher intensity of symptoms are successful with nonsurgical treatment.[65,102]

Adherence

Tendon loading exercise programs require frequent bouts of exercise for at least 3 months and adherence rates range from 72% to 100%.[103] Other treatments such as shoe inserts, medication, and TGNT also require daily adherence for effective results. The treatment plan should be discussed thoroughly with patients to optimize adherence. Particularly if tendon loading exercises are recommended, patients should be educated about expected pain responses and address their fears related to movement, which has been shown to affect treatment outcomes.[65]

Tendon Structure

Patients with greater severity of tendon pathoanatomic changes (see **Table 1**) may take longer to recover.[8,104] In addition, Achilles pathoanatomy may be impacted by compression along the medial aspect by a thickened plantaris tendon.[105]

Sensitization

Patients with AT commonly have symptoms for several months before seeking treatment.[1] Persistence of symptoms may result in central and peripheral sensitization, including secondary hyperalgesia that has been demonstrated in several tendinopathic conditions.[23] Recently, individuals with AT were found to have decreased 2-point discrimination, a sign of cortical reorganization, that may contribute to delayed or failed recovery.[22] Consideration of psychosocial and behavioral factors may be important in these patients, but further research is needed to elucidate effective management of sensitization.[23]

Table 4
Properties of PROM

Outcome Measure	Description	Reliability	MCID (Scale Points)	Cutoff Scores
VISA-A[107–109]	Specific PROM for Achilles tendon dysfunction. Includes 8 (6 visual analog and 2 categorical) response items that assesses pain, functional status, and activity domains. Scores range from 0 to 100 and higher scores indicate higher function.	Test-retest: r = 0.93 Intrarater: r = 0.90 Intrarater: r = 0.90	6.5–12	90 points = full recovery
LEFS[107,110]	Designed for a range of hip, knee, ankle, or foot conditions. Includes 20 Likert response items with a range between 0 and 80. Higher scores indicate higher function. Condition specific questionnaire for those with lower extremity musculoskeletal conditions. Each item scored on a 0–4 Likert type scale.	Test-retest: ICC = 0.86	9–12	—
FAAM[110]	Designed to assess a range of lower leg, foot, and ankle conditions. Includes a Likert response 21-item ADL and an 8-item sports subscales each scored from 0 to 100. Higher scores indicate higher function.	Test-retest: ICC = 0.87 (ADL subscale) and ICC = 0.89 (sports subscale)	ADL subscale: 8 Sports subscale: 9	—

Abbreviations: ADL, activities of daily living; ICC, intraclass correlation coefficient; FAAM, Foot and Ankle Ability Measure; LEFS, Lower Extremity Functional Scale; MCID, minimum clinically important difference; PROM, patient-reported outcome measures; VISA-A, Victorian Institute of Sport Assessment-Achilles.

EVALUATION OF OUTCOME AND LONG-TERM RECOMMENDATIONS

Recovery from AT is indicated by reduced pain and recovery of function, including a return to usual and/or recreational activities. Pain is assessed using a numeric pain rating (0–10) or visual analog scale (0–100 mm) with a 30% change indicating meaningful improvement.[106] The most widely used and valid measure of function specific to Achilles injury is the Victorian Institute of Sports Assessment-Achilles (VISA-A).[107,108] The VISA-A is a self-administered questionnaire that assesses the impact of the Achilles problem on 3 domains: (a) pain, (b) functional status, and (c) activity (**Table 4**). In addition to the VISA-A, the Foot and Ankle Ability Measure and the Lower Extremity Functional Scale are valid and reliable function scales used clinically owing to their generalizability to all foot and ankle or lower extremity conditions (see **Table 4**).

In addition to pain and function measures, biomechanical and pathoanatomic characteristics are important factors in assessing outcome and predicting long-term recovery. Musculotendon strength, endurance, and stretch-shortening cycle function were still impaired at 1 year in 75% of individuals who completed a tendon loading program despite full symptomatic and functional recovery determined by the VISA-A.[111] Therefore, heel raise or jump performance measures can be used to monitor treatment outcomes and recovery.

A lack of recovery of musculotendon function may be consistent with persistent tendon pathoanatomy. Greater tendon heterogeneity on ultrasound examination has been associated with a longer recovery time and poor outcome at 6 months of tendon loading exercise and corticosteroid injections.[8,104] Continued improvement in AT can be observed up to 1 year after starting treatment,[70] and ultrasound imaging may be useful during this time to monitor structural changes and encourage long-term adherence to tendon loading exercise. Because recovery of musculotendon function and integrity may take up to 1 year, nonsurgical management is recommended for at least 1 year (see **Fig. 2**).[65] Patients are encouraged to adhere to tendon loading exercises 2 to 3 times per week after the typical 3-month program regardless of symptomatic improvement to avoid recurrent problems related to residual biomechanical and pathoanatomic impairments.

SUMMARY

Successful management of midsubstance AT can be accomplished with nonsurgical treatment, including isolated or combined pharmacologic and nonpharmacologic treatments. Current literature supports the use of tendon loading exercise as the mainstay of chronic AT management and long-term studies (2–8 years) indicate that 80% to 90% of patients will be able to return to desired activity levels with little to no symptoms.[65,101] A variety of treatment options are used concurrently with the tendon loading program to help symptom modulation and tissue healing (see **Fig. 2**). To reduce symptoms in a reactive tendon, including acute AT, topical pharmaceuticals (iontophoresis with dexamethasone or diclofenac gel) are safe and effective solutions that avoid the risks associated with oral NSAIDs or corticosteroid injections. Other regenerative injectables (platelet-rich plasma, hypertonic glucose) have yet to demonstrate convincing evidence of effectiveness for routine use.[49] A small percentage of patients may not respond or adhere to a tendon loading program and may be candidates for shockwave or sclerosing treatment, and possibly surgery.

In addition to evidence of treatment effectiveness, intervention selection depends on clinical resources and patient preferences. Treatments such as shockwave therapy and laser may not be available in clinics near the patient.[2] Other treatments such as TGTN and sclerosing injections may require extensive and repeated application that are not conducive to the patient's circumstances. Although tendon loading exercises do not require any equipment, adherence over several months is important to achieve results and patients need to understand this fully at the outset of treatment. Patients prefer treatments with lower costs, greater chance of success, shorter time to return to their prior level of activity, and lower risks of side effects.[112] In addition, patients prefer exercises over stand-alone injections,[112] but treatment options should be discussed with each patient to identify the preferred treatment with greatest likelihood of success.

REFERENCES

1. de Jonge S, van den Berg C, de Vos RJ, et al. Incidence of midportion Achilles tendinopathy in the general population. Br J Sports Med 2011;45(13):1026–8.
2. Rowe V, Hemmings S, Barton C, et al. Conservative management of midportion Achilles tendinopathy: a mixed methods study, integrating systematic review and clinical reasoning. Sports Med 2012;42(11):941–67.
3. Silbernagel KG, Crossley KM. A proposed return-to-sport program for patients with midportion Achilles tendinopathy: rationale and implementation. J Orthop Sports Phys Ther 2015;45(11):876–86.
4. Franettovich Smith MM, Honeywill C, Wyndow N, et al. Neuromotor control of gluteal muscles in runners with Achilles tendinopathy. Med Sci Sports Exerc 2014;46(3):594–9.
5. Azevedo LB, Lambert MI, Vaughan CL, et al. Biomechanical variables associated with Achilles tendinopathy in runners. Br J Sports Med 2009;43(4):288–92.
6. Alfredson H, Lorentzon R. Chronic Achilles tendinosis: recommendations for treatment and prevention. Sports Med 2000;29(2):135–46.
7. Cook JL, Purdam CR. Is tendon pathology a continuum? A pathology model to explain the clinical presentation of load-induced tendinopathy. Br J Sports Med 2009;43(6):409–16.
8. Bakkegaard M, Johannsen FE, Højgaard B, et al. Ultrasonography as a prognostic and objective parameter in Achilles tendinopathy: a prospective observational study. Eur J Radiol 2015;84(3):458–62.
9. Astrom M, Gentz CF, Nilsson P, et al. Imaging in chronic Achilles tendinopathy: a comparison of ultrasonography, magnetic resonance imaging and surgical findings in 27 histologically verified cases. Skeletal Radiol 1996;25(7):615–20.
10. Sconfienza LM, Silvestri E, Cimmino MA. Sonoelastography in the evaluation of painful Achilles tendon in amateur athletes. Clin Exp Rheumatol 2010;28(3):373–8.
11. De Zordo T, Chhem R, Smekal V, et al. Real-time sonoelastography: findings in patients with symptomatic Achilles tendons and comparison to healthy volunteers. Ultraschall Med 2010;31(4):394–400.
12. De Jonge S, Warnaars JLF, De Vos RJ, et al. Relationship between neovascularization and clinical severity in Achilles tendinopathy in 556 paired measurements. Scand J Med Sci Sports 2014;24(5):773–8.
13. Kaufman KR, Brodine SK, Shaffer RA, et al. The effect of foot structure and range of motion on musculoskeletal overuse injuries. Am J Sports Med 1999;27(5):585–93.
14. Mahieu NN, Witvrouw E, Stevens V, et al. Intrinsic risk factors for the development of Achilles tendon overuse injury: a prospective study. Am J Sports Med 2006;34(2):226–35.
15. McCrory JL, Martin DF, Lowery RB, et al. Etiologic factors associated with Achilles tendinitis in runners. Med Sci Sports Exerc 1999;31(10):1374–81.

16. Ryan M, Grau S, Krauss I, et al. Kinematic analysis of runners with Achilles mid-portion tendinopathy. Foot Ankle Int 2009;30(12):1190–5.

17. Clement DB, Taunton JE, Smart GW. Achilles tendinitis and peritendinitis: etiology and treatment. Am J Sports Med 1984;12(3):179–84.

18. Alfredson H, Pietila T, Jonsson P, et al. Heavy-load eccentric calf muscle training for the treatment of chronic Achilles tendinosis. Am J Sports Med 1998;26(3):360–6.

19. Silbernagel KG, Gustavsson A, Thomee R, et al. Evaluation of lower leg function in patients with Achilles tendinopathy. Knee Surg Sports Traumatol Arthrosc 2006;14(11):1207–17.

20. Arya S, Kulig K. Tendinopathy alters mechanical and material properties of the Achilles tendon. J Appl Physiol (1985) 2010;108(3):670–5.

21. Child S, Bryant AL, Clark RA, et al. Mechanical properties of the Achilles tendon aponeurosis are altered in athletes with Achilles tendinopathy. Am J Sports Med 2010;38(9):1885–93.

22. Debenham J, Butler P, Mallows A, et al. Disrupted tactile acuity in people with achilles tendinopathy: a preliminary case-control investigation. J Orthop Sports Phys Ther 2016. http://dx.doi.org/10.2519/jospt.2016.6514.

23. Plinsinga ML, Brink MS, Vicenzino B, et al. Evidence of nervous system sensitization in commonly presenting and persistent painful tendinopathies: a systematic review. J Orthop Sports Phys Ther 2015;45(11):864–75.

24. Holmes GB, Lin J. Etiologic factors associated with symptomatic Achilles tendinopathy. Foot Ankle Int 2006;27(11):952–9.

25. Ames PRJ, Longo UG, Denaro V, et al. Achilles tendon problems: not just an orthopaedic issue. Disabil Rehabil 2008;30(20–22):1646–50.

26. Gaida JE, Alfredson L, Kiss ZS, et al. Dyslipidemia in Achilles tendinopathy is characteristic of insulin resistance. Med Sci Sports Exerc 2009;41(6):1194–7.

27. Reiman M, Burgi C, Strube E, et al. The utility of clinical measures for the diagnosis of Achilles tendon injuries: a systematic review with meta-analysis. J Athl Train 2014;49(6):820–9.

28. Jan M-H, Chai H-M, Lin Y-F, et al. Effects of age and sex on the results of an ankle plantar-flexor manual muscle test. Phys Ther 2005;85(10):1078–84.

29. Martin RL, McPoil TG. Reliability of ankle goniometric measurements: a literature review. J Am Podiatr Med Assoc 2005;95(6):564–72.

30. McPoil TG, Cornwall MW, Vicenzino B, et al. Effect of using truncated versus total foot length to calculate the arch height ratio. Foot (Edinb) 2008;18(4):220–7.

31. Redmond AC, Crosbie J, Ouvrier RA. Development and validation of a novel rating system for scoring standing foot posture: the Foot Posture Index. Clin Biomech 2006;21(1):89–98.

32. Redmond AC, Crane YZ, Menz HB. Normative values for the foot posture index. J Foot Ankle Res 2008;1(1):6.

33. Carcia CR, Martin RL, Houck J, et al. Association, orthopaedic section of the American physical therapy. Achilles pain, stiffness, and muscle power deficits: Achilles tendinitis. J Orthop Sports Phys Ther 2010;40(9):A1–26.

34. Piva SR, Fitzgerald K, Irrgang JJ, et al. Reliability of measures of impairments associated with patellofemoral pain syndrome. BMC Musculoskelet Disord 2006;7:33.

35. de Jonge S, Tol JL, Weir A, et al. The tendon structure returns to asymptomatic values in nonoperatively treated Achilles tendinopathy but is not associated with symptoms: a prospective study. Am J Sports Med 2015;43(12):2950–8.

36. Maffulli N, Papalia R, D'Adamio S, et al. Pharmacological interventions for the treatment of Achilles tendinopathy: a systematic review of randomized controlled trials. Br Med Bull 2015;113(1):101–15.
37. Knobloch K. Tendinopathy and drugs–potential implications for beneficial and detrimental effects on painful tendons. J Sci Med Sport 2009;12(3):423.
38. Asplund CA, Best TM. Achilles tendon disorders. BMJ 2013;346:f1262.
39. Corrao G, Zambon A, Bertù L, et al. Evidence of tendinitis provoked by fluoroquinolone treatment. Drug Saf 2006;29(10):889–96.
40. Kim GK. The risk of fluoroquinolone-induced tendinopathy and tendon rupture: what does the clinician need to know? J Clin Aesthet Dermatol 2010;3(4):49–54.
41. Alfredson H, Cook J. A treatment algorithm for managing Achilles tendinopathy: new treatment options. Br J Sports Med 2007;41(4):211–6.
42. Paoloni JA, Milne C, Orchard J, et al. Non-steroidal anti-inflammatory drugs in sports medicine: guidelines for practical but sensible use. Br J Sports Med 2009;43(11):863–5.
43. Magra M, Maffulli N. Nonsteroidal antiinflammatory drugs in tendinopathy: friend or foe. Clin J Sport Med 2006;16(1):1–3.
44. Åström M, Westlin N. No effect of piroxicam on Achilles tendinopathy: a randomized study of 70 patients. Acta Orthop Scand 1992;63(6):631–4.
45. Andres BM, Murrell GAC. Treatment of tendinopathy: what works, what does not, and what is on the horizon. Clin Orthop Relat Res 2008;466(7):1539–54.
46. Ziltener JL, Leal S, Fournier PE. Non-steroidal anti-inflammatory drugs for athletes: an update. Ann Phys Rehabil Med 2010;53(4):278–88.
47. Paoloni JA, Murrell GAC. Three-year followup study of topical glyceryl trinitrate treatment of chronic noninsertional Achilles tendinopathy. Foot Ankle Int 2007;28(10):1064–8.
48. Paoloni JA, Appleyard RC, Nelson J, et al. Topical glyceryl trinitrate treatment of chronic noninsertional Achilles tendinopathy. A randomized, double-blind, placebo-controlled trial. J Bone Joint Surg Am 2004;86-A(5):916–22.
49. Kearney RS, Parsons N, Metcalfe D, et al. Injection therapies for Achilles tendinopathy. Cochrane Database Syst Rev 2015;(5):CD010960.
50. Neeter C, Thomeé R, Silbernagel KG, et al. Iontophoresis with or without dexamethasone in the treatment of acute Achilles tendon pain. Scand J Med Sci Sports 2003;13(6):376–82.
51. Fredberg U, Bolvig L, Pfeiffer-Jensen M, et al. Ultrasonography as a tool for diagnosis, guidance of local steroid injection and, together with pressure algometry, monitoring of the treatment of athletes with chronic jumper's knee and Achilles tendinitis: a randomized, double-blind, placebo-controlled study. Scand J Rheumatol 2004;33(2):94–101.
52. DaCruz DJ, Geeson M, Allen MJ, et al. Achilles paratendonitis: an evaluation of steroid injection. Br J Sports Med 1988;22(2):64–5.
53. Loveless MS, Fry AL. Pharmacologic therapies in musculoskeletal conditions. Med Clin North Am 2016;100(4):869–90.
54. Derry S, Moore RA, Gaskell H, et al. Topical NSAIDs for acute musculoskeletal pain in adults. Cochrane Database Syst Rev 2015;(6):CD007402.
55. Argoff CE. Topical analgesics in the management of acute and chronic pain. Mayo Clin Proc 2013;88(2):195–205.
56. Nourissat G, Ornetti P, Berenbaum F, et al. Does platelet-rich plasma deserve a role in the treatment of tendinopathy? Joint Bone Spine 2015;82(4):230–4.
57. Moraes VY, Lenza M, Tamaoki MJ, et al. Platelet-rich therapies for musculoskeletal soft tissue injuries. Cochrane Database Syst Rev 2014;(4):CD010071.

58. Metcalfe D, Achten J, Costa ML. Glucocorticoid injections in lesions of the Achilles tendon. Foot Ankle Int 2009;30(7):661–5.
59. Magnussen RA, Dunn WR, Thomson AB. Nonoperative treatment of midportion Achilles tendinopathy: a systematic review. Clin J Sport Med 2009;19(1):54–64.
60. Alfredson H, Ohberg L. Sclerosing injections to areas of neo-vascularisation reduce pain in chronic Achilles tendinopathy: a double-blind randomised controlled trial. Knee Surg Sports Traumatol Arthrosc 2005;13(4):338–44.
61. Ohberg L, Alfredson H. Ultrasound guided sclerosis of neovessels in painful chronic Achilles tendinosis: pilot study of a new treatment. Br J Sports Med 2002;36(3):173–5 [discussion: 176–177].
62. Lind B, Ohberg L, Alfredson H. Sclerosing polidocanol injections in mid-portion Achilles tendinosis: remaining good clinical results and decreased tendon thickness at 2-year follow-up. Knee Surg Sports Traumatol Arthrosc 2006;14(12): 1327–32.
63. van Sterkenburg MN, de Jonge MC, Sierevelt IN, et al. Less promising results with sclerosing ethoxysclerol injections for midportion Achilles tendinopathy a retrospective study. Am J Sports Med 2010;38(11):2226–32.
64. Alfredson H. Clinical commentary of the evolution of the treatment for chronic painful mid-portion Achilles tendinopathy. Braz J Phys Ther 2015;19(5):429–32.
65. Silbernagel KG, Brorsson A, Lundberg M. The majority of patients with Achilles tendinopathy recover fully when treated with exercise alone: a 5-year follow-up. Am J Sports Med 2011;39(3):607–13.
66. Habets B, van Cingel REH. Eccentric exercise training in chronic mid-portion Achilles tendinopathy: a systematic review on different protocols. Scand J Med Sci Sports 2015;25(1):3–15.
67. Rompe JD, Nafe B, Furia JP, et al. Eccentric loading, shock-wave treatment, or a wait-and-see policy for tendinopathy of the main body of tendo Achillis: a randomized controlled trial. Am J Sports Med 2007;35(3):374–83.
68. Roos EM, Engström M, Lagerquist A, et al. Clinical improvement after 6 weeks of eccentric exercise in patients with mid-portion Achilles tendinopathy – a randomized trial with 1-year follow-up. Scand J Med Sci Sports 2004;14(5):286–95.
69. Stevens M, Tan C-W. Effectiveness of the Alfredson protocol compared with a lower repetition-volume protocol for midportion Achilles tendinopathy: a randomized controlled trial. J Orthop Sports Phys Ther 2014;44(2):59–67.
70. Silbernagel KG, Thomeé R, Eriksson BI, et al. Continued sports activity, using a pain-monitoring model, during rehabilitation in patients with Achilles tendinopathy: a randomized controlled study. Am J Sports Med 2007;35(6):897–906.
71. Silbernagel KG, Thomeé R, Thomeé P, et al. Eccentric overload training for patients with chronic Achilles tendon pain–a randomised controlled study with reliability testing of the evaluation methods. Scand J Med Sci Sports 2001;11(4): 197–206.
72. Beyer R, Kongsgaard M, Hougs Kjær B, et al. Heavy slow resistance versus eccentric training as treatment for Achilles tendinopathy: a randomized controlled trial. Am J Sports Med 2015;43(7):1704–11.
73. Couppé C, Svensson RB, Silbernagel KG, et al. Eccentric or concentric exercises for the treatment of tendinopathies? J Orthop Sports Phys Ther 2015; 45(11):853–63.
74. Malliaras P, Barton CJ, Reeves ND, et al. Achilles and patellar tendinopathy loading programmes : a systematic review comparing clinical outcomes and identifying potential mechanisms for effectiveness. Sports Med 2013;43(4): 267–86.

75. Mayer F, Hirschmuller A, Muller S, et al. Effects of short-term treatment strategies over 4 weeks in Achilles tendinopathy. Br J Sports Med 2007;41(7):e6.

76. Donoghue OA, Harrison AJ, Laxton P, et al. Orthotic control of rear foot and lower limb motion during running in participants with chronic Achilles tendon injury. Sports Biomech 2008;7(2):194–205.

77. Wyndow N, Cowan SM, Wrigley TV, et al. Neuromotor control of the lower limb in Achilles tendinopathy: implications for foot orthotic therapy. Sports Med 2010; 40(9):715–27.

78. Chimenti RL, Flemister AS, Ketz J, et al. Ultrasound strain mapping of Achilles tendon compressive strain patterns during dorsiflexion. J Biomech 2016; 49(1):39–44.

79. Stergioulas A, Stergioula M, Aarskog R, et al. Effects of low-level laser therapy and eccentric exercises in the treatment of recreational athletes with chronic Achilles tendinopathy. Am J Sports Med 2008;36(5):881–7.

80. Tumilty S, McDonough S, Hurley DA, et al. Clinical effectiveness of low-level laser therapy as an adjunct to eccentric exercise for the treatment of Achilles' tendinopathy: a randomized controlled trial. Arch Phys Med Rehabil 2012; 93(5):733–9.

81. Vicenzino B. Foot orthotics in the treatment of lower limb conditions: a musculoskeletal physiotherapy perspective. Man Ther 2004;9(4):185–96.

82. Smith M, Brooker S, Vicenzino B, et al. Use of anti-pronation taping to assess suitability of orthotic prescription: case report. Aust J Physiother 2004;50(2): 111–3.

83. Firth BL, Dingley P, Davies ER, et al. The effect of kinesiotape on function, pain, and motoneuronal excitability in healthy people and people with Achilles tendinopathy. Clin J Sport Med 2010;20(6):416–21.

84. Lee J-H, Yoo W-G. Treatment of chronic Achilles tendon pain by Kinesio taping in an amateur badminton player. Phys Ther Sport 2012;13(2):115–9.

85. Lim ECW, Tay MGX. Kinesio taping in musculoskeletal pain and disability that lasts for more than 4 weeks: is it time to peel off the tape and throw it out with the sweat? A systematic review with meta-analysis focused on pain and also methods of tape application. Br J Sports Med 2015;49(24):1558–66.

86. McCormack JR. The management of mid-portion Achilles tendinopathy with astym(R) and eccentric. Int J Sports Phys Ther 2012;7(6):672–7.

87. Miners AL, Bougie TL. Chronic Achilles tendinopathy: a case study of treatment incorporating active and passive tissue warm-up, Graston Technique, ART, eccentric exercise, and cryotherapy. J Can Chiropr Assoc 2011;55(4):269–79.

88. Papa JA. Conservative management of Achilles Tendinopathy: a case report. J Can Chiropr Assoc 2012;56(3):216–24.

89. Simons DG, Travell JG, Simons LS. Travell & Simons' myofascial pain and dysfunction: the trigger point manual. 2nd edition. Baltimore: Williams & Wilkins; 1999.

90. Nørregaard J, Larsen CC, Bieler T, et al. Eccentric exercise in treatment of Achilles tendinopathy. Scand J Med Sci Sports 2007;17(2):133–8.

91. Welsh RP, Clodman J. Clinical survey of Achilles tendinitis in athletes. Can Med Assoc J 1980;122(2):193–5.

92. Kane TP, Ismail M, Calder JD. Topical glyceryl trinitrate and noninsertional Achilles tendinopathy: a clinical and cellular investigation. Am J Sports Med 2008; 36(6):1160–3.

93. Rasmussen S, Christensen M, Mathiesen I, et al. Shockwave therapy for chronic Achilles tendinopathy: a double-blind, randomized clinical trial of efficacy. Acta Orthop 2008;79(2):249–56.

94. Mani-Babu S, Morrissey D, Waugh C, et al. The effectiveness of extracorporeal shock wave therapy in lower limb tendinopathy: a systematic review. Am J Sports Med 2015;43(3):752–61.

95. Knobloch K, Schreibmueller L, Longo UG, et al. Eccentric exercises for the management of tendinopathy of the main body of the Achilles tendon with or without the AirHeelTM Brace. A randomized controlled trial. A: effects on pain and microcirculation. Disabil Rehabil 2008;30(20–22):1685–91.

96. Eliasson P, Andersson T, Aspenberg P. Achilles tendon healing in rats is improved by intermittent mechanical loading during the inflammatory phase. J Orthop Res 2012;30(2):274–9.

97. Matsumoto F, Trudel G, Uhthoff HK, et al. Mechanical effects of immobilization on the Achilles' tendon. Arch Phys Med Rehabil 2003;84(5):662–7.

98. Trudel G, Koike Y, Ramachandran N, et al. Mechanical alterations of rabbit Achilles' tendon after immobilization correlate with bone mineral density but not with magnetic resonance or ultrasound imaging. Arch Phys Med Rehabil 2007;88(12):1720–6.

99. de Jonge S, de Vos RJ, Van Schie HTM, et al. One-year follow-up of a randomised controlled trial on added splinting to eccentric exercises in chronic midportion Achilles tendinopathy. Br J Sports Med 2010;44(9):673–7.

100. de Vos RJ, Weir A, Visser RJA, et al. The additional value of a night splint to eccentric exercises in chronic midportion Achilles tendinopathy: a randomised controlled trial. Br J Sports Med 2007;41(7):e5.

101. Ohberg L, Lorentzon R, Alfredson H. Eccentric training in patients with chronic Achilles tendinosis: normalised tendon structure and decreased thickness at follow up. Br J Sports Med 2004;38(1):8–11 [discussion: 11].

102. Paavola M, Kannus P, Paakkala T, et al. Long-term prognosis of patients with Achilles tendinopathy. An observational 8-year follow-up study. Am J Sports Med 2000;28(5):634–42.

103. Sussmilch-Leitch SP, Collins NJ, Bialocerkowski AE, et al. Physical therapies for Achilles tendinopathy: systematic review and meta-analysis. J Foot Ankle Res 2012;5(1):15.

104. Archambault JM, Wiley JP, Bray RC, et al. Can sonography predict the outcome in patients with achillodynia? J Clin Ultrasound 1998;26(7):335–9.

105. Masci L, Spang C, van Schie HTM, et al. How to diagnose plantaris tendon involvement in midportion Achilles tendinopathy - clinical and imaging findings. BMC Musculoskelet Disord 2016;17(1):97.

106. Dworkin RH, Turk DC, Wyrwich KW, et al. Interpreting the clinical importance of treatment outcomes in chronic pain clinical trials: IMMPACT recommendations. J Pain 2008;9(2):105–21.

107. McCormack J, Underwood F, Slaven E, et al. The minimum clinically important difference on the VISA-A and LEFS for patients with insertional Achilles tendinopathy. Int J Sports Phys Ther 2015;10(5):639–44.

108. Robinson JM, Cook JL, Purdam C, et al. The VISA-A questionnaire: a valid and reliable index of the clinical severity of Achilles tendinopathy. Br J Sports Med 2001;35(5):335–41.

109. Iversen JV, Bartels EM, Langberg H. The Victorian Institute of Sports Assessment - Achilles questionnaire (VISA-A) - a reliable tool for measuring Achilles tendinopathy. Int J Sports Phys Ther 2012;7(1):76–84.

110. Martin RL, Irrgang JJ. A survey of self-reported outcome instruments for the foot and ankle. J Orthop Sports Phys Ther 2007;37(2):72–84.
111. Silbernagel KG, Thomee R, Eriksson BI, et al. Full symptomatic recovery does not ensure full recovery of muscle-tendon function in patients with Achilles tendinopathy. Br J Sports Med 2007;41(4):276–80 [discussion: 280].
112. Sweeting KR, Whitty JA, Scuffham PA, et al. Patient preferences for treatment of Achilles tendon pain: results from a discrete-choice experiment. Patient 2011; 4(1):45–54.

Midsubstance Tendinopathy, Percutaneous Techniques (Platelet-Rich Plasma, Extracorporeal Shock Wave Therapy, Prolotherapy, Radiofrequency Ablation)

William Bret Smith, DO, MSc*, Will Melton, MD, James Davies, MD

KEYWORDS

- Achilles • Percutaneous • Alternative treatment • Injections • Ultrasound

KEY POINTS

- Noninsertional Achilles tendinopathy has been addressed with numerous treatment algorithms ranging from physiotherapy to surgery.
- Percutaneous treatments are commonly advocated as an intermediate modality between surgery and conservative management.
- Percutaneous techniques have wide variability in administration and efficacy.

INTRODUCTION

Achilles noninsertional tendinopathy can be a challenging pathophysiology to treat. The typical initial treatment phase tends to focus on a combination of rest, activity modifications, therapy protocols, and possible protective devices. At the opposite end of the treatment spectrum would be numerous surgical options. Occasionally, the authors have patients with symptoms and pathologic conditions that may be amenable to an intermediary treatment option, that is, percutaneous techniques. Because the proposed mechanism for degeneration of the noninsertional region of the Achilles has been purported by some researchers to be decreased local microvascular circulation,[1] many of the proposed treatments on the percutaneous arm focus on opportunities to promote the body's ability to repair damaged tissue. Whether the

Department of Orthopedics, University of South Carolina, 2 Medical Park, Columbia, SC, USA
* Corresponding author.
E-mail address: wbsmithdo@yahoo.com

Clin Podiatr Med Surg 34 (2017) 161–174
http://dx.doi.org/10.1016/j.cpm.2016.10.005
0891-8422/17/© 2017 Elsevier Inc. All rights reserved.

theories on ischemic change are the primary pathophysiologic cause of the condition or whether it is mechanically based degeneration has been debated. Similar debates exist regarding the mechanisms by which these different modalities provide relief. Ultimately the goal of most percutaneous procedures is to stimulate a healing response from the body in the damaged tendon tissue.

Percutaneous treatment protocols offer a very attractive option and have garnered significant interest in the orthopedic community. Because they are by design minimally invasive, they are attractive to many providers with the goal of minimizing risk related to open procedures. The evidence regarding the efficacy of these procedures is varied with a lot of anecdotal and industry recommendations discussed. As with any new treatment modality, we must continue to critically analyze the research to determine if the efficacy and cost-effectiveness warrant its consideration for treatment in our patients. The focus of this article is to present the current options available for noninvasive and percutaneous treatment options for noninsertional Achilles tendinopathy. An attempt is made to offer recommendations for both the treatment techniques as well as postprocedure protocols to be considered. Additionally, because there are numerous treatment options in this category, the different techniques are summarized in chart format with a short list of pros and cons as well as the levels of evidence in the literature to support the different modalities (**Table 1**).

INDICATIONS

Generally, indications for percutaneous treatment of midsubstance tendinopathy represent an area between failed conservative treatment and surgical treatment (**Box 1**). Conservative treatment usually involves eccentric stretching, rest and activity medication, shoe modification and inserts, and nonsteroidal medication. Extracorporeal shock wave therapy (ECSWT), prolotherapy, platelet-rich plasma (PRP), and radiofrequency ablation (RF) can be used as an adjunct to these treatment modalities. ECSWT,[2–5] prolotherapy,[6–10] and RF[11,12] can be used for pain management. ECSWT has also been reported to improve functional outcomes.[2–5]

Furthermore, if patients are not surgical candidates, these treatments offer another option. ECSWT, prolotherapy, and RF theoretically improve vascularity leading to a more robust healing response. This increased vascularity could counter the known pathologic conditions of midsubstance tendinopathy preventing further surgical intervention. If patients progress, then the increased blood flow at that site could facilitate incision and soft tissue healing. This healing could potentially improve outcomes for patients with known factors that predispose to tendinopathy as well as poor wound healing, including diabetes mellitus, obesity, and steroid use.[13]

General contraindications are related to the need for surgical intervention. A large partial tear or a full tear typically necessitates surgical intervention. Failure of conservative therapy has been correlated with severity of tendon degeneration, age, and duration of symptoms.[14] Although no definitive timetable has been established, studies have noted a duration greater than 6 months as well as greater than 8 to 12 weeks as more likely to lead to surgical intervention.[15,16]

As ECSWT has been a treatment option for years, there is extensive research advocating its use. During this time, specific contraindications have been recommended, including pregnancy, coagulopathies, osseous tumors, osseous infections, and skeletal immaturity.[17] RF is a relatively newer treatment modality; but, in a 2012 study by Shibuya and colleagues,[18] 3 of 47 patients experienced a rupture following RF. All 3 had a high body mass index (BMI). However, the investigators noted mild trauma

Table 1
Tendinopathy literature review summary

Treatment Modality	Advantages	Disadvantages	Best Level of Evidence
Platelet-rich plasma	• Shown to be beneficial in combination with eccentric exercises • Relatively inexpensive compared with surgical intervention ($500–$800) • Safe/relatively low risk associated with injection	• Not shown to be more effective than eccentric exercise alone • Variability of postoperative protocols • Variable results with conflicting methodologies & inconclusive evidence	Level I–IV
Extracorporeal shock wave therapy	• Shown to be beneficial in combination with eccentric exercises • Often twice the cost of platelet-rich plasma but still inexpensive compared with surgical intervention • Viable treatment option after other treatments have failed and before considering surgical intervention for Achilles tendinopathy	• Not shown to be more effective than eccentric exercise alone • High dose damages neovasculature and surrounding tissue • Tendon rupture reported as complication in some studies • Inconsistent definition of low-high ECSWT • Multiple techniques to generate pulses • Recommend against use in pregnancy, coagulopathy, infection, skeletal immaturity	Level I–IV
Prolotherapy	• Relatively inexpensive ($300–$400) • Safe/relatively low risk associated with injection • Good option for patients with high surgical risk	• Not shown to be more effective than eccentric exercise on higher-evidence studies • No well-defined standard prolotherapy concentration or duration of treatments	Level I–IV
Radiofrequency	• Improved angiogenesis in animal model • Improved clinical outcomes from 6 mo to 3 y in smaller studies • Good option for patients with high surgical risk	• Most studies showed radiofrequency ablation treatment required general anesthesia or intravenous sedation • Low levels of evidence • Increased BMI associated with complications including tendon rupture • Study results convoluted by concomitant procedures • No good long-term studies • More expensive than other modalities	Level IV–V
TENEX	• Very low reported complication rates • Small studies report excellent results	• Very limited data • Low levels of evidence • Studies and data from single centers • No good long-term studies • More expensive than other modalities	Level IV–V

> **Box 1**
> **Indications**
>
> 1. Adjunct to conservative treatment
> 2. Failed conservative treatment
>   - Delayed presentation
>   - Prolonged duration
> 3. Poor surgical candidate
>   - Poor wound healing potential
>   - High anesthetic risk

associated with the rupture obscuring the correlation with obesity. There were no specific contraindications for PRP or prolotherapy in regard to midsubstance tendinopathy reported in the literature (**Table 2**).

COMPLICATIONS

Because of the paucity of clinical research, there are few documented complications from these techniques. There were no reported complications of PRP injection or prolotherapy injection found in the literature,[19] but there are possible complications for any injection.[19] For RF, there has been documented tendon rupture in 3 cases in the study previously mentioned as well as one case report for insertional tendinopathy in 2009.[20] The reported and theoretic complications are listed:

- ECSWT
  - Dose dependent[17]
    - Low dose is safer than high dose
    - High dose damages neo-vasculature and surrounding tissue
  - Tendon rupture reported in 2 patients[21]
    - Unclear if related to treatment
  - Mild, transient skin erythema[21]
- PRP
  - Related to injection
    - Injury to blood vessel
    - Sural nerve injury
- Prolotherapy
  - Related to injection
    - Injury to blood vessel
    - Sural nerve injury
- RF
  - Tendon rupture

Table 2 Contraindications	
1. Needs surgical intervention	• Present for >6 mo (relative duration) • Large defect or rupture
2. ECSWT	• Pregnancy • Coagulopathy • Bone tumor or infection • Skeletal maturity
3. RF	• High BMI (relative)

PLATELET-RICH PLASMA OUTCOMES

Recent literature attempted to validate a role for PRP in the treatment of chronic mid-substance Achilles tendinopathy and concluded the patients who received PRP injection demonstrated modest improvement in functional outcome measures; however, MRI appearance of diseased Achilles tendons remained largely unchanged following PRP injection.[22,23] Patients underwent a single PRP injection for the treatment of chronic midsubstance Achilles tendinopathy and were evaluated at a 6-month final follow-up. A retrospective evaluation of patients receiving a single PRP injection for chronic midsubstance Achilles tendinopathy revealed that 78% had experienced clinical improvement and had avoided surgical intervention at the 6-month follow-up.[24]

A stratified, block-randomized, double-blind, placebo-controlled trial at a single center (The Hague Medical Center, Leidschendam, the Netherlands) of 54 randomized patients aged 18 to 70 years with chronic tendinopathy 2 to 7 cm above the Achilles tendon insertion. Among patients with chronic Achilles tendinopathy who were treated with eccentric exercises, a PRP injection compared with a saline injection did not result in greater improvement in pain and activity.[25]

Another double-blinded, randomized, placebo-controlled clinical trial set out to assess whether a PRP injection led to an enhanced tendon structure and neovascularization, measured with ultrasonography techniques, in chronic midportion Achilles tendinopathy. The study concluded injecting PRP for the treatment of chronic midportion Achilles tendinopathy did not contribute to an increased tendon structure or alter the degree of neovascularization, compared with placebo.[26]

Overall, a systematic review of the available literature concluded that the literature surrounding injectable treatments for noninsertional Achilles tendinosis including PRP have variable results with conflicting methodologies and inconclusive evidence concerning indications for treatment and the mechanism of their effects on chronically degenerated tendons.[27,28] These inconclusive results were again demonstrated in a randomized, blinded, placebo-controlled trail in 2016 that showed no difference between the PRP and the saline group could be observed in terms of outcomes.[28,29]

Platelet-Rich Plasma Procedure

Multiple PRP preparation methods are available; the injection amounts, concentrations, and the number of injections vary between studies. Concentration of platelets in PRP can vary from 2.5 to 9.0 times that of normal.[6] In one randomized controlled trial, PRP injection was prepared using the recover platelet separation kit, in accordance with the system instructions.[12] Fifty-four milliliters of venous blood was collected from the cubital vein. The whole blood was mixed with 6 mL of citrate to prevent early clotting. After blood collection and 15 minutes of centrifugation, PRP was obtained. To match the pH of PRP with the pH of the tendon tissue, 0.3 mL of 8.4% sodium bicarbonate buffer was added. PRP was injected under ultrasonography control. An average volume of 3 mL PRP was injected into the hypoechogenic areas of affected tendons.[22]

Preprocedure Planning

Clinical diagnosis can be confirmed with either ultrasonography or MRI. Some investigators suggest discontinuing nonsteroidal antiinflammatory drugs (NSAIDs) up to 2 weeks before injection.

Prep and Patient Positioning

Prone, lateral positioning is used.

POSTPROCEDURE CARE

Decision making about postoperative care and weight-bearing status is hindered by the diversity of published works and should be based on both surgeon preference/ discretion and area and quality of tendon tissue. After the initial procedure, patients can be placed into a removable walker boot. Postinjection protocols vary substantially in the published literature, and the current authors are unable to make definitive recommendations on the most efficacious postinjection protocol after a thorough literature review.

Several randomized controlled trials have used the following postoperative protocol or one very similar following PRP injection: Patients were advised to avoid full loading of the limb, to use elbow crutches, and to elevate the limb for 3 days after injection. In the next 2 weeks, patients used walking crutches with pressure applied on the anterior section of the foot and passively exercised the ankle joint. For the subsequent 2 weeks, the load on the foot was increased using a heel lift in the patients' own shoes; passive exercises and active exercises without load were continued. Six weeks after injection, full load without crutches began.[22]

The following postinjection protocol has also been suggested:

- For the first 2 to 3 days adhere to the following: no weight bearing and elevation, no activity, and rest only.
- On day 3 to 4, remove the boot throughout the day to work on full range of motion without resistance and begin to transition out of the boot for walking as able over the next 1 to 2 weeks.
- On day 4 to 14, begin resistance eccentric exercise with the limb: 2 sets of 30 gentle repetitions twice a day. Gradually increase resistance. It is vital to move the limb to stimulate proper healing. Cardiovascular exercise can be maintained with such activities as walking, swimming, upper-body bike, recumbent bike, elliptical, and so forth.
- Formal physical therapy can begin at 2 weeks.

EXTRACORPOREAL SHOCK WAVE THERAPY OUTCOMES

A recent systematic review and meta-analysis aimed to assess the short-term (<12 months) and long-term (>12 months) effectiveness of ECSWT in treating Achilles tendinopathy. The energy level, number of impulses, number of sessions, and use of a local anesthetic varied between studies. Additionally, current evidence is limited by low participant numbers and several methodological weaknesses, including inadequate randomization. Moderate evidence indicates that ECSWT is more effective than eccentric loading for insertional achilles tendinopathy (AT) and equal to eccentric loading for mid-portion AT in the short term. Additionally, there is moderate evidence that combining ECSWT and eccentric loading in mid-portion AT may produce superior outcomes to eccentric loading alone.[30]

The 2 randomized controlled trials of ECSWT suggest that it may be of utility in the treatment of chronic midportion Achilles tendinopathy. These trials use low- to medium-energy ECSWT (0.1–0.2 mJ/mm^2) without the use of general anesthesia.[4,31]

In one study, patients were blinded to the treatment they received, and the treatment effect was not significant.[4,21,31] A recent randomized controlled trial investigating high-energy ECSWT for insertional Achilles tendinopathy showed significant pain relief at 1 year.[32] Investigation of the effect of ECSWT therapy for tendinopathy in other anatomic locations has been extensive and contradictory, with numerous randomized trials showing success as well as multiple randomized trials failing to show an effect.[2–4,21,31–37] In another randomized controlled trail, at the 4-month follow-up, eccentric loading alone was less effective when compared with a combination of eccentric loading and repetitive low-energy shock-wave treatment.[31] Interpretation of these data is complicated by the inconsistent definition of low- and high-energy ECSWT and the use of multiple techniques to generate the pulses. Clear definition of terms and consistent technique will be necessary in future randomized controlled trials in this area.[31]

Procedure

Decision making about whether to use ECSWT and the energy levels, number of treatment sessions, and number of impulses to choose is hindered by the diversity of published works. The benefits of using a local anesthetic are also disputed but can be used before each treatment. The procedure lasts approximately 30 to 45 minutes. One published study reported using 3000 shocks: 0.21 mJ/mm^2, total energy flux density, 604 mJ/mm.[31]

Preprocedure Planning

Clinical diagnosis can be confirmed with either ultrasonography or MRI.

Prep and Patient Positioning

Positioning can be prone, lateral, or seated depending on the design of the ECSWT method being used.

Postprocedure Care

Decision making about postoperative care and weight bearing status is hindered by the diversity of published works and lack of any defined consensus, Postoperative protocols can range from immobilization and non–weight bearing to using a walker boot with or without heel wedges for full weight bearing. This depends on individual surgeon preference and discretion and should be based on pathologic conditions and amount of tissue treated. Postinjection protocols vary substantially in the published literature, and the current authors are unable to make definitive recommendations on the most efficacious posttreatment protocol after a thorough literature review.

PROLOTHERAPY OUTCOMES

Although smaller studies have shown prolotherapy to be a safe, effective, and inexpensive treatment of Achilles tendinopathy,[6] and also improved outcomes when combined with eccentric exercises,[10] recent level 1 evidence in a systematic review found limited evidence that prolotherapy injections are an effective treatment of Achilles tendinopathy. This review noted that although most patients in previously reported trials reported sustained improvements in pain, stiffness and overall satisfaction, there were few statistically or clinically significant differences between groups; other studies did not find any benefit to prolotherapy alone in the absence of eccentric exercises.[10,19] A 2010 meta-analysis did not demonstrate that prolotherapy was more effective than eccentric exercises.[38,39]

Smaller studies comparing the effectiveness and cost-effectiveness of eccentric loading exercises with prolotherapy injections used singly and in combination for painful Achilles tendinosis found that for Achilles tendinosis, prolotherapy and particularly eccentric loading exercises combined with prolotherapy gave more rapid improvements in symptoms than eccentric loading exercises alone but long-term improvement scores are similar.[10,19]

Although numerous smaller studies claim to demonstrate prolotherapy as an effective option, numerous level I evidence studies; both systematic reviews, and meta-analyses like have found no increased benefit. Incomplete reporting of study quality and small sample sizes means that the reviewers' conclusions, although cautious, may not be reliable.[40]

Procedure

Prolotherapy injection preparations have been described: a standard solution of 20% dextrose and 0.1% lignocaine administered weekly along the affected tendon. It is hypothesized that injection of dextrose causes local cell necrosis as a direct result of osmotic shock.[38] Thought to work via "therapeutic trauma" at the injection site initiates the body's wound healing cascade of inflammation, granulation tissue formation, and matrix formation and remodeling.[41–43] In one randomized trial, the physician injected tender points in the subcutaneous tissues adjacent to the affected Achilles tendon with a solution consisting of 20% glucose/0.1% lignocaine/0.1% ropivacaine weekly for 4 to 12 treatments, using the technique described by Lyftogt[6]; the number of treatments was determined by the time it took to reach a pain-free activity or until the participant requested to cease treatment.[10] In the Lyftogt[6] study, the prolotherapy (PrT) group received injections of solution consisting of 50% dextrose, 5% sodium morrhuate, 4% lidocaine, and 0.5% bupivacaine hydrochloride (Sensorcaine). The study pharmacists mixed the following: 35.0 mL sterile solution, 7.5 mL 50% dextrose, 5.0 mL 5% sodium morrhuate, 2.5 mL 4% lidocaine, 2.5 mL 0.5% Sensorcaine, and 17.5 mL normal saline. The solution was 10.7% dextrose and contained 14.7% sodium morrhuate by volume. Using a 25-gauge 1.5-in needle, the lead investigator injected 0.5 mL.[6] No defined prolotherapy preparation concentration is favored in the literature. The physician may choose to use topical analgesia if desired.

Preprocedure Planning

Clinical diagnosis can be confirmed with either ultrasonography or MRI.

Prep and Patient Positioning

Positioning is the physicians' preference.

Postprocedure Care

Overall, postinjection protocols may be managed similarly to those for post-PRP injection; but as with PRP injection also, decision making about postoperative care and weight-bearing status is hindered by the diversity of published works, and injection protocols vary substantially in the published literature. Postoperative protocols can range from immobilization and non–weight bearing to using a walker boot with or without heel wedges for full weight bearing.

The current authors are unable to make definitive recommendations on the most efficacious postinjection protocol after a thorough literature review.

RADIOFREQUENCY ABLATION OUTCOMES

A recent 2012 review of 47 cases with percutaneous radiofrequency coblation techniques was conducted and demonstrated surprisingly high numbers of complications in terms of requiring further intervention, which was alarming at 14.9% (7 of 47). Rupture of the Achilles tendon was identified in 3 (6.4%) patients. Complication rate seemed associated with higher BMIs.[18]

Other small studies using bipolar radiofrequency microtenotomy in the treatment of Achilles tendonitis reported good short-term outcomes and pain relief at 6 months,[12] and another study's results over 3 years have demonstrated 90% to 95% good to excellent results.[44]

A study conducted using a rabbit model reported an increase in the expression of the angiogenic markers, alpha-v and vascular endothelial growth factor, in tendons treated with bipolar radiofrequency coblation, suggesting that such an application may provide a viable option where angiogenesis is important to the outcome, such as Achilles tendonitis.[45,46]

Other radiofrequency study results are convoluted by combining radiofrequency techniques with concomitant procedures, such as fascial incision, adhesiolysis, arthroscopy, or tendoscopy. Long-term, randomized, double-blind studies are still needed.

Procedure

Coblation-based technology operates at low temperature (40°C–70°C) unlike other radiofrequency-based surgical products, such as laser and electro-surgical devices, which use a heat-driven process. Coblation technology is a controlled, non–heat-driven process that uses radiofrequency energy to excite the electrolytes in a conductive medium, such as saline solution, creating a precisely focused charged plasma gas. The energized particles in plasma have sufficient energy to break the molecular bonds within tissue, causing tissue to dissolve at relatively low temperatures.[47]

In one review of 47 cases, local infiltrative anesthesia was placed proximal to the area of treatment after either general anesthesia or intravenous sedation. The agent used for local anesthesia varied between the surgeons. No surgeon used a vasoconstrictive agent or intraoperative cortisone. The operative extremity was then prepped in a usual sterile fashion, and the tourniquet was inflated to an appropriate level. Using a marking pen, dots were made over the posterior aspect of the Achilles tendon, covering the point of maximum tenderness. Approximately 20 points were mapped out, and an 18-gauge needle was used to make small holes through the skin. The radiofrequency probe (Topaz Microdebrider; ArthroCare, Sunnyvale, CA) was then used to perform the procedure, hole by hole, via a controlled plasma-mediated radiofrequency-based process. The probe was activated for 0.5 seconds while light axial pressure was applied to puncture the tendon perpendicularly. No skin closure was performed. Sterile dressings were placed over the operative site. The patient was placed in an immobilization boot and allowed full weight bearing immediately.[18]

Preprocedure Planning

Clinical diagnosis can be confirmed with either ultrasonography or MRI. It is suggested to refrain from NSAID use beginning 2 weeks before procedure.

Prep and Patient Positioning

It is usually prone.

Postprocedure Care

Decision making about postoperative care and weight-bearing status is hindered by the diversity of published works and the extent of the RF tissue debridement but can range from immobilization and non–weight bearing to using a walker boot with or without heel wedges for full weight bearing.[18]

Some investigators suggest refraining from NSAID use up to 6 weeks following the procedure.

The patients were encouraged to ice and elevate the operated extremity for the first 2 to 3 days. NSAIDs were not allowed for the first 48 hours. The first postoperative visit was 3 to 5 days from the surgery, and a surgical dressing change was performed during the visit. Although this varied slightly between the surgeons, the second post-operative visit was at approximately 2 weeks, at which point the patients began range-of-motion exercises and eccentric stretching exercises but remained in the immobilization boot for weight bearing. At the 1-month follow-up visit, the patients were transitioned to regular shoe gear and continued the exercises. After approximately 3 months, the patients were generally released to return to full activities as tolerated.[18]

Another study in which RF was used through a small incision discussed the following postoperative protocol.[47]

- 3 weeks non–weight bearing in a posterior splint or fiberglass cast
- Followed by 3 to 6 weeks weight bearing in a pneumatic CAM walker
- 6 weeks postoperatively, patients are able to begin range of motion and physical therapy
- 6 to 8 weeks postoperatively patients return to their normal show wear

TENEX OUTCOMES

Results at present are small in number and have primarily focused on elbow tendon-itis; but it is, nevertheless, being promoted for the Achilles with very little depth of data for support. A recent investigation prospectively documented the safety and 1-year ef-ficacy of ultrasonic percutaneous tenotomy of the elbow performed by a single oper-ator. No procedural complications occurred. The results in this small study demonstrated that percutaneous ultrasonic tenotomy performed under local anes-thesia seems to be a safe and effective treatment option for chronic, refractory lateral or medial elbow tendinopathy up to 1 year after the procedure.[48] Another recent study in 2013 also reported improved clinical outcomes at 1 year, but again this was shown for lateral elbow tendinopathy.[49]

Another study found minimally invasive percutaneous ultrasonic tenotomy provided sustained pain relief and functional improvement for recalcitrant tennis elbow at the 3-year follow-up.[49] It is one of the few procedures to demonstrate positive sono-graphic evidence of tissue-healing response and is an attractive alternative to surgical intervention for definitive treatment of recalcitrant elbow tendinopathy.[50]

Although its utilization in Achilles tendinopathy has been limited in the literature, initial results are encouraging. A 2013 study of TENEX on a subset of the rabbits with collagenase induced Achilles tendinosis were exposed to an ultrasound-guided percutaneous tenotomy. Histopathologic examination at 3 weeks revealed that, in an-imals treated with the TENEX System, expression of collagens I, III, and X returned to levels similar to a normal tendon. In conclusion, these results are encouraging for the use of the TENEX System as a definitive treatment of chronic tendinopathic lesions, based on the cutting and removal of degraded tendon material.[51]

A recent retrospective review reported on 26 consecutive patients (7 male/21 fe-male) with chronic insertional tendinopathy who underwent percutaneous tenotomy using the ultrasonic percutaneous tenotomy. The patients had failed an average of 5.8 (range 4–8) conservative treatments over an average period of 18 months. Patients were evaluated 1 week, 1 month, and periodically up to 16 months after the procedure. Of the 26 patients treated, 23 (88.5%) described pain relief from the procedure and 24 (92.3%) would have the procedure done again or recommend the procedure.[52]

Overall, the literature is considerably limited on the application of ultrasonic percutaneous tenotomy for Achilles tendinopathy, and further investigation is warranted.

Procedure

In the office setting, using ultrasound guidance to target the exact location of pain and tendinopathy, a local anesthetic, such as lidocaine, is used to numb the area. Ultrasound imaging is used to identify the area of scar tissue again, and the physician inserts the toothpick-sized tip of the TENEX Tissue Removal System into the affected tendon. The tip emits ultrasonic energy, which cuts and breaks down damaged, painful scar tissue without disturbing the surrounding healthy tendon tissue. It has also been reportedly used for removal of small osteophytes and bone spurs. Tenex Health TX is referred to as focused aspiration of scar tissue and is performed with a microtip (which consists of an 18-gauge needle within an irrigation sheath that is calibrated to debride scar and pathologic tissue and not healthy tendon tissue). Again, it is suggested that this be done under ultrasound guidance.[53,54]

For a recently published prospective study on percutaneous ultrasonic tenotomy using TENEX for chronic elbow tendinosis: guidelines were total treatment time less than 15 minutes, and ultrasonic energy time averaged 38.6 ± 8.8 seconds per procedure.[48] Ultimately, the procedure time will vary depending on degree and area of tendinopathy.

Preprocedure Planning

Clinical diagnosis can be confirmed with either ultrasonography or MRI.

Prep and Patient Positioning

Patients are preferably placed prone or lateral.

Postprocedure Care

Decision making about postoperative care and weight-bearing status is hindered by the lack of published/available literature and should be based on both surgeon preference/discretion and area and quality of tendon tissue. After the initial procedure, patients can be placed into a removable walker boot or initial splint. A recovery period has been suggested as a 1- to 2-month timeframe before return to full activities.[53]

SUMMARY

Currently, there is no evidence that PRP injections provide statistically significant relief versus placebo in multiple randomized trials.[25,29,55–57] Therefore, routine use for midsubstance Achilles tendinopathy cannot be recommended at this time. There has been evidence to support the use of ECSWT, prolotherapy, and RF as adjuncts to conservative therapy when conservative therapy has failed or when patients are poor surgical candidates. However, there is also evidence of no changes in pain[21,25] and no changes in function[21] for ECSWT. This finding underscores the need for more research, specifically more research with a strong study design. This point has been well documented in multiple systematic reviews.[28,58,59] Further research with consistent treatment methods and standardization of protocols could provide more evidence for these minimally invasive options.

REFERENCES

1. Kujala UM, Sarana S, Kaprio J. Cumulative incidence of Achilles tendon rupture and tendinopathy in male former elite athletes. Clin J Sport Med 2005;15(3): 133–5.
2. Lakshmanan P, O'Doherty D. Chronic Achilles tendinopathy: treatment with extracorporeal shock waves. Foot Ankle Surg 2004;10(3):125–30.
3. Rompe J, Furia J, Maffuli N. Mid-portion Achilles tendinopathy: current options for treatment. Disabil Rehabil 2008;30(20–22):1666–76.
4. Rompe J, Nafe B, Furia J, et al. Eccentric loading, shock-wave treatment, or a wait-and-see policy for tendinopathy of the main body of tendo Achilles: a randomized controlled trial. Am J Sports Med 2007;35(3):347–83.
5. Vulpiani M, Trischitta D, Trovato P, et al. Extracorporeal shockwave therapy (ESWT) in Achilles tendinopathy: a long-term follow-up observational study. J Sports Med Phys Fitness 2009;49(2):171–6.
6. Lyftogt J. Prolotherapy and Achilles tendinopathy: a prospective pilot study of an old treatment. Australasian Musculoskeletal Medicine 2005;10:16–9.
7. Lyftogt J. Subcutaneous prolotherapy for Achilles tendinopathy: the best solution? Australasian Musculoskeletal Medicine 2007;12(2):107–9.
8. Maxwell N, Ryan M, Taunton J, et al. Sonographically guided intratendinous injection of hyperosmolar dextrose of the Achilles tendon: a pilot study. Am J Roentgenol 2007;189(4):215–20.
9. Ryan M, Wong A, Taunton J. Favorable outcomes after sonographically guided intratendinous injection of hyperosmolar dextrose for chronic insertional and midpoint Achilles tendinosis. AJR Am J Roentgenol 2010;194:1047–53.
10. Yellend M, Sweeting K, Lyftogt J, et al. Prolotherapy injections and eccentric loading exercises for painful Achilles tendinosis: a randomized trial. Br J Sports Med 2011;45:421–8.
11. Liu Y, Wang Z, Li Z, et al. Arthroscopically assisted radiofrequency probe to treat Achilles tendinitis. Zhonghua Wai Ke Za Zhi 2008;46(2):101–3.
12. Yeap E, Chong K, Yeo W, et al. Radiofrequency coblation for chronic foot and ankle tendinosis. J Orthop Surg (Hong Kong) 2009;17(3):325–30.
13. Holmes G, Lin J. Etiologic factors associated with symptomatic Achilles tendinopathy. Foot Ankle Int 2006;27:952–9.
14. Alfredson H, Cook J. A treatment algorithm for managing Achilles tendinopathy: new treatment options. Br J Sports Med 2007;41:211–6.
15. Kvist H, Kvist M. The operative treatment of chronic calcaneal paratenonitis. J Bone Joint Surg Br 1980;62(3):353–7.
16. Schepsis A, Wagner C, Leach R. Surgical management of Achilles tendon overuse injuries. A long-term follow-up study. Am J Sports Med 1994;22(5):611–9.
17. Chung B, Wiley P. Extracorporeal shockwave therapy: a review. Sports Med 2002; 32(13):851–65.
18. Shibuya N, Thorus J, Humphers J, et al. Is percutaneous radiofrequency coblation for treatment of Achilles tendinosis safe and effective? J Foot Ankle Surg 2012;51:767–71.
19. Sanderson L, Bryant A. Effectiveness and safety of prolotherapy injections for management of lower limb tendinopathy and fasciopathy: a systemic review. J Foot Ankle Res 2015;8:60.
20. Akhtar M, Montgomery H, Shenolikar A. Achilles tendon rupture following coblation for insertional Achilles tendinosis. Foot (Edinb) 2009;19(1):55–7.

21. Costa M, Shepstone L, Donnell S, et al. Shock wave therapy for chronic Achilles tendon pain: a randomized controlled trial. Clin Orthop Relat Res 2005;440: 199–204.
22. Gaweda K, Tarczynska M, Krzyzanowski W. Treatment of Achilles tendinopathy with platelet-rich plasma. Int J Sports Med 2010;31(8):577–83.
23. Owen R, Conti S, Ginnetti J, et al. Clinical and magnetic resonance imaging outcomes following platelet rich plasma injection for chronic midsubstance Achilles tendinopathy. Foot Ankle Int 2011;32(11):1032–9.
24. Murawski CD, Smyth NA, Newman H, et al. A single platelet-rich plasma injection for chronic midsubstance Achilles tendinopathy: a retrospective preliminary analysis. Foot Ankle Spec 2014;7(5):372–6.
25. de Vos RJ, Weir A, van Schie HT, et al. Platelet-rich plasma injection for chronic Achilles tendinopathy: a randomized controlled trial. JAMA 2010;303(2):144–9.
26. de Vos RJ, Weir A, Tol JL, et al. No effects of PRP on ultrasonographic tendon structure and neovascularisation in chronic midportion Achilles tendinopathy. Br J Sports Med 2011;45(5):387–92.
27. AHRQ Healthcare Horizon Scanning System potential high impact interventions: priority area 01: arthritis and nontraumatic joint disease. Agency for Healthcare Research and Quality. Available at: https://www.effectivehealthcare.ahrq.gov/ehc/assets/File/01_Arthritis_Potential_High_Impact_2012-12-10.pdf.
28. Gross C, Hsu A, Chahal J, et al. Injectable treatments for noninsertional Achilles tendinosis: a systematic review. Foot Ankle Int 2013;34(5):619–28.
29. Krogh T, Ellingsen T, Christensen R, et al. Ultrasound-guided injection therapy of Achilles tendinopathy with platelet-rich plasma or saline: a randomized, blinded, placebo-controlled trial. Am J Sports Med 2016;44(8):1990–7.
30. Mani-Babu S, Morrissey D, Waugh C, et al. The effectiveness of extracorporeal shock wave therapy in lower limb tendinopathy: a systematic review. Am J Sports Med 2015;43(3):752–61.
31. Magnussen RA, Dunn WR, Thomson AB. Nonoperative treatment of midportion Achilles tendinopathy: a systematic review. Clin J Sport Med 2009;19(1):54–64.
32. Furia JP. High-energy extracorporeal shock wave therapy as a treatment for chronic noninsertional Achilles tendinopathy. Am J Sports Med 2008;36(3):502–8.
33. Buchbinder R, Ptasznik R, Gordon J, et al. Ultrasound-guided extracorporeal shock wave therapy for plantar fasciitis: a randomized controlled trial. JAMA 2002;288:1364–72.
34. Haake M, Konig IR, Decker T, et al. Extracorporeal shock wave therapy in the treatment of lateral epicondylitis: a randomized multicenter trial. J Bone Joint Surg Am 2002;84-A:1982–91.
35. Speed CA, Nichols D, Richards C, et al. Extracorporeal shock wave therapy for lateral epicondylitis–a double blind randomised trial. J Orthop Res 2002;20:895–8.
36. Hammer DS, Rupp S, Kreutz A, et al. Extracorporeal shockwave therapy (ESWT) in patients with chronic proximal plantar fasciitis. Foot Ankle Int 2002;23:309–13.
37. Langer P. Two emerging technologies for Achilles tendinopathy and plantar fasciopathy. Clin Podiatr Med Surg 2015;32:183–93.
38. Coombes BK, Bisset L, Vicenzino B. Efficacy and safety of corticosteroid injections and other injections for management of tendinopathy: a systematic review of randomised controlled trials. Lancet 2010;376(9754):1751–67.
39. O'Brien M. Functional anatomy & physiology of tendons. Clin Sports Med 1992; 11:505–20.
40. Centre for Reviews & Dissemination. A systematic review of four injection therapies for lateral epicondylosis: DARE commentary on 2009 review by Rabago

et al. DARE (Database of Abstracts of Reviews of Effects) 2010. Available at: https://www.crd.york.ac.uk/CRDWeb/ResultsPage.asp.

41. Harvey M. Prolotherapy for podiatrists–part 1, understanding dense connective tissue [Internet]. Chiropody Review. 2011. Available at: http://www.aspc-uk.net/wp-content/uploads/2014/03/Prolotherapy-for-Podiatrists-part-1-understanding-dense-connective-tissue.pdf. Accessed September 4, 2014.

42. Freeman J, Empson Y, Ekwueme E, et al. Effect of prolotherapy on cellular proliferation and collagen deposition in MC3T3-E1 and patellar tendon fibroblast populations. Transl Res 2011;158:132–9.

43. Martins C, Bertuzzi R, Tisot R, et al. Dextrose prolotherapy and corticosteroid injection into rat Achilles tendon. Knee Surg Sports Traumatol Arthrosc 2012; 20(10):1895–900.

44. Tasto JP. The use of bipolar radiofrequency microtenotomy in the treatment of chronic tendinosis of the foot and ankle. Tech Foot Ankle Surg 2006;5(2):110–6.

45. Harwood F, Bowden K, Ball S, et al. Structural and angiogenic response to bipolar radiofrequency treatment of normal rabbit Achilles tendon. Trans Orthop Res Soc 2003;28:819.

46. Roche C. A review of the current concepts of treatment: Achilles tendinopathy. Bone Joint J 2013;95-B(10):1299–307.

47. Brosky T, Thomas J. Topaz coblation of Achilles tendon pathology. The Podiatry Institute Update; 2007. Available at: https://www.podiatryinstitute.com/textbooks.htm.

48. Barnes MD, Beckley MD, Smith MD. Percutaneous ultrasonic tenotomy for chronic elbow tendinosis: a prospective study. J Shoulder Elbow Surg 2015;24(1):67–73.

49. Koh JS, Mohan PC, Howe TS, et al. Fasciotomy and surgical tenotomy for recalcitrant lateral elbow tendinopathy: early clinical experience with a novel device for minimally invasive percutaneous microresection. Am J Sports Med 2013;41(3):636–44.

50. Seng C, Mohan PC, Koh SB, et al. Ultrasonic percutaneous tenotomy for recalcitrant lateral elbow tendinopathy: sustainability and sonographic progression at 3 years. Am J Sports Med 2016;44(2):504–10.

51. Kamineni S, Butterfield T, Sinai A. Percutaneous ultrasonic debridement of tendinopathy – a pilot Achilles rabbit model. J Orthop Surg Res 2015;10:70.

52. Ellis M, Johnson K, Freed L, et al. Fasciotomy and surgical tenotomy for chronic Achilles insertional tendinopathy: a retrospective study using ultrasound-guided percutaneous tenotomy approach. J Am Podiatr Med Assoc, in press.

53. Available at: https://www.tenexhealth.com/. Accessed August, 2015.

54. Available at: http://www.herrerasportsmedicine.com/tenex-health-procedure-elbow-knee-shoulder-tendinitis.html. Accessed August, 2015.

55. de Jong S, de Vos R, Weir A, et al. One-year follow-up of platelet-rich plasma treatment in chronic Achilles tendinopathy: a double-blind randomized placebo–controlled trial. Am J Sports Med 2001;39:1623–9.

56. Rasmussen S, Christensen M, Mathiesen I, et al. Shockwave therapy for chronic Achilles tendinopathy: a double-blind, randomized clinical trial of efficacy. Acta Orthop 2008;79(2):249–56.

57. Guelfi M, Pantalone A, Vanni D, et al. Long-term beneficial effects of platelet-rich plasma for non-insertional Achilles tendinopathy. Foot Ankle Surg 2015;21(3): 178–81.

58. Al-Abbad H, Simon J. The effectiveness of extracorporeal shock wave therapy on chronic Achilles tendinopathy: a systematic review. Foot Ankle Int 2012;34(1):33–41.

59. Maxwell N, Ryan MB, Taunton JE, et al. Sonographically guided intratendinous injection of hyperosmolar dextrose to treat chronic tendinosis of the Achilles tendon: a pilot study. AJR Am J Roentgenol 2007;189:w215–20.

Midsubstance Tendinopathy, Surgical Management

William T. DeCarbo, DPM[a],*, Mark J. Bullock, DPM[b]

KEYWORDS

- Noninsertional achilles • Achilles peritendinitis • Achilles paratendinopathy
- Achilles tendinosis • Achilles tendinopathy • Flexor hallucis longus transfer

KEY POINTS

- For an athlete with isolated paratendinopathy, open paratenon release/excision and ventral paratenon scraping have high reported success rates.
- If a core area of tendinopathy is present, longitudinal excision is the treatment of choice.
- Minimally invasive techniques have lower wound complication rates but require further study.
- A flexor hallucis longus (FHL) tendon transfer or turndown flap can supplement the repair when there is extensive tendinopathy.
- Gastrocnemius recession has higher reported success rates in the treatment of noninsertional Achilles tendinopathy compared with insertional Achilles tendinopathy.

INTRODUCTION (NATURE OF THE PROBLEM)

Midsubstance Achilles tendinopathy is a commonly seen painful condition of the Achilles tendon located in the area approximately 2 cm to 7 cm proximal to its calcaneal insertion. The literature discussing Achilles dysfunction and terminology can be confusing and contradictory. Terms, such as tenosynovitis, paratenonitis, peritendinitis, paratendinitis, paratendinopathy, tendinitis, tendinosis, tendinopathy, and achillodynia, have all been associated with noninsertional Achilles pain.[1] It is often described as an overuse injury seen in athletes and older individuals, with a higher male predilection.[2–4] The incidence varies from 0.2% in the general population, up to 9% in recreational runners.[5,6] Symptoms include pain, swelling, and impaired performance. Maffulli and colleagues[7] noted this pathology often includes histologic findings of tendinosis and paratendinopathy.

Disclosure Statement: The authors have nothing to disclose.
[a] The Orthopedic Group, 800 Plaza Drive, Suite 240, Belle Vernon, PA 15012, USA; [b] Saginaw Valley Bone and Joint Center, 5483 Gratiot Road, Saginaw, MI 48638, USA
* Corresponding author.
E-mail address: wdecarbo@yahoo.com

Having an anatomic understanding of the posterior leg and calf is essential in understanding Achilles pathology. The anatomic, histologic, and vascular structure has been well described in the literature and is discussed in detail (see Paul Dayton's article, "Anatomic, Vascular and Mechanical Overview of the Achilles Tendon," in this issue).[8–16] The clinical presentation of Achilles pain differs in location between posterior heel pain at the back of the foot, insertional tendinopathy, pain in the Achilles tendon at the back of the leg, and noninsertional tendinopathy. Patients with insertional heel pain have pain and edema at the posterior calcaneus. This usually hurts in shoes from the heel counter and hurts with palpation. This too is usually exacerbated with physical activity. Enthesopathy or calcification within the tendon at its insertion is commonly appreciated. Care must be taken to differentiate noninsertional Achilles tendinopathy from the subset of insertional Achilles tendinopathy caused by Haglunds deformity because Achilles impingement lesions can extend to the watershed region (**Fig. 1**).

For noninsertional Achilles tendinopathy, patients present with pain in the back of the Achilles area usually with a bump (**Fig. 2**). Often patients relate a history of nonsignificant trauma, such as a sprain, twisting, or "overdoing it." The pain typically progresses over time and seems to hurt with increased activity before patients seek medical treatment. Lateral radiographs may reveal calcifications within the tendon (**Fig. 3**).

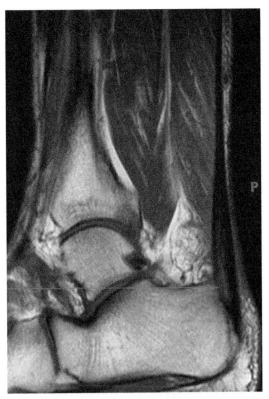

Fig. 1. MRI showing Achilles impingement tendinopathy in contact with Haglund deformity. Achilles lesion on the ventral side of the tendon extends to the watershed area.

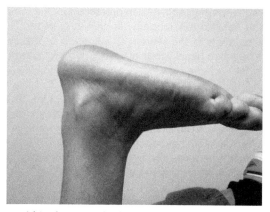

Fig. 2. Bulbous mass within the watershed area is appreciated on physical examination.

A patient's history provides useful information to aid in the diagnosis of Achilles tendinopathy. Onset of symptoms, recent or previous injuries to the Achilles tendon, and previous treatment are keys for making a diagnosis.[17] Patients in an early phase complain of pain after strenuous activity whereas those who complain of pain during and after any activity are in a later phase. Those in the later phase

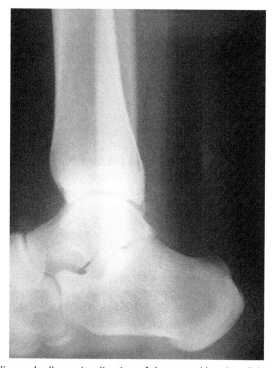

Fig. 3. Lateral radiograph allows visualization of the ventral border of the tendon along Kager triangle. The Achilles tendon is thickened in the watershed area with extensive calcifications.

typically do not tolerate sporting activity. On presentation, the most common symptom of a patient with Achilles tendinopathy is pain. It is imperative to pinpoint the precise location of pain within the tendon.[17] Palpation of a bulbous mass within the tendon or at its insertion usually indicates a more chronic pathology (tendinopathy) whereas diffuse edema and erythema may indicate an acute onset (paratendinopathy).[18]

Differential diagnosis may include fracture, bursitis, rupture of the posterior tibial tendon, neurologic disorders, calcaneal periostitis, Haglund syndrome, Sever disease, bone disorders, compartment syndrome, plantar fasciitis, muscle strains, or other soft tissue problems. Systemic diseases, such as rheumatoid or inflammatory arthritis, seronegative spondyloarthropathies, Reiter syndrome, infection, metabolic disorders, and connective tissue disease must also be considered.[19]

Radiographs should be taken with special attention paid to the lateral and calcaneal axial films. Ultrasonography has proved a quick, accurate, and inexpensive modality in observing intratendinous lesions or thickening of the Achilles.[20] This is operator dependent and less sensitive, however, than MRI.[21] Fluid may be observed around the tendon in the acute setting, while chronically hypoechoic areas within the tendon or paratenon with fibrous disruptions representing adhesions may be noted.[22] MRI is the most common and reliable imaging modality to examine the Achilles tendon. Not only does it allow for detailed 3-D imaging of anatomic structures but also it distinguishes between normal and abnormal tissue. Imaging often reveals thickening of the tendon with intratendinous signal abnormalities.[21] Disadvantages of MRI include high cost and a time-consuming scanning process.[23]

Achilles tendinopathy on a histopathologic level can be divided into 2 findings: peritendinous changes and intratendinous degeneration, which often coexist.[24] In chronic Achilles tendinopathy, peritendinous changes observed include an abundance of fibroblasts and myofibroblasts, where myofibroblasts synthesize collagen, causing adhesions. Intratendinous degenerative changes, as described by Åström and Rausing,[3] is characterized by vascular proliferation, presence of fibrinogen, focal hypercellularity, and abnormal fiber structure in the symptomatic parts of the tendon. Hypervascularity, macrophages, and fibroblasts may represent a failed healing response. The etiology of tendinopathy is poorly understood with repetitive overload, hypoxia, free radicals, and persistent inflammation proposed as sources for Achilles tendon degeneration.[22]

The concept of neovascularizaton is an area of ongoing research for midsubstance Achilles tendinopathy. Neovascularization is the ingrowth of vasculature and sensory neurons into the ventral Achilles tendon in response to Achilles injury. Patients with chronic midsubstance Achilles tendinopathy have been shown to have increased blood flow along the ventral Achilles tendon on color Doppler compared with controls.[25] Additionally, patients with biopsies of chronic Achilles tendinopathy have increased sensory neurons that stain with substance P compared with patients who had acute ruptures with no prior symptoms.[26] In the patellar tendon, tendinopathy was associated with increased substance P sensory neurons compared with asymptomatic controls.[27] It is not known whether the degree of neovascularization correlates with the severity of symptoms because the literature has shown inconsistent results.[28–32] Neovascularization is the basis behind procedures that release and/or scrape the ventral paratenon.

Initially, treatment of midsubstance Achilles tendinopathy is conservative. Conservative treatment of noninsertional Achilles tendinopathy is focused around rest and activity modification. If a patient presents with a lot of pain, a tall walking boot is used as first-line treatment to calm down the tendon. The walking boot is used until the initial presenting symptoms are decreased or resolved, usually 1 to 2 weeks. Concomitantly nonsteroidal anti-inflammatorie drugs (NSAIDs) are started to help with patient discomfort. NSAIDs have been shown to have a modest effect in treating tendinopathy but their use is questionable due to the histologic absence of inflammatory cells with chronic tendinopathy.[32–35] The short-term benefit related to use of NSAIDs is most likely due to the analgesic effect of these medications.[36]

Corticosteroid injections have been used with much controversy. Reports have shown a decrease in pain and swelling[7,37] but there is a high complication rate reported, including risk of acute tendon rupture.[38] Any benefit gained from corticosteroid injections is outweighed by the potential risks, and this treatment is not recommended by the authors.[39]

The mainstay for long-term relief of symptoms with noninsertional Achilles tendinopathy is centered on physical therapy with eccentric exercises of the Achilles tendon.[40–42] The mechanical loading of the Achilles tendon with eccentric exercises increases the fluctuations in applied force compared with concentric exercises [43] Alfredson and colleagues[44] performed a randomized study comparing eccentric and concentric exercises over a 12-week program. The investigators reported that 82% of patients in the eccentric exercise group returned to normal activities at 12 weeks compared with only 36% in the concentric group. The results were also sustained over a 12-month period[45]; 6-week programs with eccentric exercises have also shown efficacy.[46–48] Compliance may be a cause of failure when patients undergo an eccentric training program. A recent randomized controlled trial (RCT) found patients undergoing slow resistance training had a higher satisfaction rate at 12 weeks compared with eccentric training, 100% versus 80%. Patients in the slow resistance training group were found to have a higher compliance rate, 96% versus 76%.[49]

Extracorporeal shockwave therapy for the treatment of noninsertional Achilles tendinopathy has also been described with conflicting results.[50,51] The authors have no direct experience with this treatment modality.

Platelet-rich plasma (PRP) has been used to treat a wide variety of orthopedic pathologies in recent years, with significant improvement of symptoms when used in tendon therapy.[52–55] Unfortunately, these same results have not been reported when using PRP for Achilles tendinopathy.[52,56] de Vos and colleagues[57] performed a randomized double-blind placebo-controlled study evaluating eccentric exercises and PRP or saline injections for Achilles tendinopathy. The study showed no difference in improvement in pain and activity at 6 months between the 2 groups. Sadoghi and colleagues[58] recently concluded PRP may be beneficial in increasing healing strength with acute Achilles tendon ruptures; however, there is no evidence showing benefit in using PRP in the treatment of Achilles tendinopathy.

The degree of tendon degeneration and thickening may be a cause for failure of conservative treatment. This finding has been reported for insertional Achilles tendinopathy but it has not been studied in noninsertional Achilles tendinopathy to the authors' knowledge.[59] The degree of tendon degeneration on ultrasound also correlates with the risk of acute Achilles tendon rupture with tendons greater than 8 mm in diameter on ultrasound having a high risk of rupture.[60] The authors prefer conservative treatment — initial rest, activity modification, and if needed walking boot mobilization. NSAIDs are offered as well. After the initial pain/discomfort is calmed down, aggressive eccentric loading of the Achilles tendon is initiated. Stretching is accomplished with a night splint, home stretching exercises, and physical therapy.

INDICATIONS/CONTRAINDICATIONS

Surgery is indicated in the treatment of noninsertional Achilles tendinopathy after failure of an eccentric exercise program for 3 to 6 months.[22] Surgery may be considered earlier if there is risk of rupture with anteroposterior tendon diameter greater than 8 mm.[60]

Surgery for noninsertional Achilles tendinopathy is elective and is contraindicated in the presence of severe peripheral vascular disease, abnormal coagulation tests, or active infection.

SURGICAL TECHNIQUE/PROCEDURE (PREOPERATIVE, PREPARATION/POSITION, SURGICAL APPROACH, AND SURGICAL PROCEDURE)
Achilles Side-to-Side Repair

Surgical treatment of midsubstance Achilles tendinopathy is reserved for cases that fail exhaustive conservative treatment. Noninsertional surgical repair is focused around débridement of all tendinopathy or nonviable tendon. This débridement is thought to initiate vascular ingrowth and a healing response.[33,61] The authors' preferred operative treatment is an open technique with the patient in a prone position. A posterior medial incision is made over the area of the diseased tendon extending distally and proximally approximately 3 cm beyond the zone of tendinopathy (**Fig. 4**). Alternatively, a posterior central incision can be used to preserve the angiosomes of the posterior leg.[62] Sharp dissection is carried out through the paratenon (**Fig. 5**). Care is made to not layer dissect this area with the medial and lateral skin flaps providing full-thickness flaps. No-touch technique is used with minimal retraction. Usually retraction with your opposite hand is adequate to separate the tissue.

The area of Achilles tendinopathy is identified, which is usually bulbous and slightly discolored from the surrounding tendon. The devitalized tendon is débrided longitudinally with 2 converging semielliptical incisions extending through the tendon full thickness from posterior to anterior (**Fig. 6**). The diseased tendon is removed and passed off to the back table. The remaining tendon is inspected for any remaining diseased or nonviable tissue. The débrided tendon is then repaired with tubularization of the anterior portion of the tendon (**Fig. 7**) followed by the posterior portion usually with a running interlocking suture technique (**Fig. 8**). This is accomplished with either 0 or 2-0 gauge absorbable or nonabsorbable suture. The authors prefer 0 Vicryl for both deep and superficial repair.

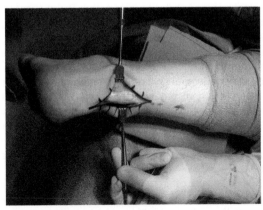

Fig. 4. Incision over the Achilles tendon is made just medial to midline to avoid the sural nerve.

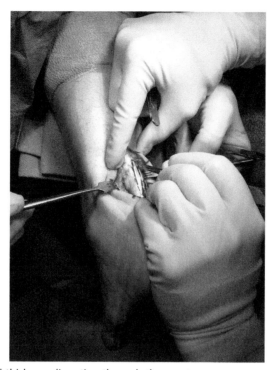

Fig. 5. Sharp, full-thickness dissection through the paratenon.

The subcutaneous tissue and skin are closed accordingly in 1 full-thickness layer usually with 2-0 absorbable suture. Skin is closed with either staples or sutures based on surgeon preference. A dry sterile bulky dressing is applied with the limb placed into a gravity equinus posterior splint.

Flexor Hallucis Longus Tendon Transfer

For Achilles tendinopathy where débridement is greater than 50% of the tendon, it has been recommended to augment the Achilles with a neighboring tendon transfer (**Fig. 9**). The FHL tendon is the most commonly used. The FHL tendon has many advantages with transfer. It fires in the same phase of gait as the Achilles, is in close proximity, has good vascularity, and is the second strongest plantarflexor.[63] DeCarbo and Hyer[64] described a single incision short harvest with interference screw fixation. This obviates a plantar medial foot incision. Peroneus brevis tendon and flexor digitorum longus tendon have also been described to augment the Achilles with both having disadvantages and are not as ideal as the FHL tendon.[63,65] Nunley and colleagues[66] reported 96% satisfaction with good function at 7 years with no augmentation.

When a tendon transfer augmentation is deemed appropriate, the authors prefer using the FHL tendon. The same surgical approach is made with the tendinopathy débrided full thickness, as described previously. With the Achilles débrided/split longitudinally, access to the posterior deep fascia and the FHL tendon muscle belly is readily available. Access can often be gained either through the split Achilles approach to the posterior compartment or by retracting the débrided Achilles laterally.

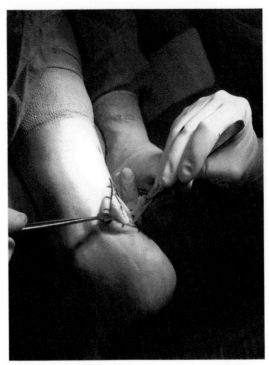

Fig. 6. Discolored, thickened tendinopathy is excised as a longitudinal ellipse through the full thickness of the Achilles tendon.

Once the tendon is retracted, sharp dissection through the posterior deep fascia is carried out exposing the FHL tendon muscle belly and tendon complex. The FHL tendon muscle tendon junction is identified and retracted out of the incision with a blunt retractor or a finger (**Fig. 10**). The FHL tendon sheath is released into the porta pedis of the foot with careful retraction of the neurovascular structures, which lie just anterior and medial to the tendon. Once the tendon is isolated, blunt retraction pulling the tendon out of the incision is performed with the ankle and hallux in maximum plantarflexion to gain as much length of the FHL tendon as possible. With the neurovascular structures protected, the FHL tendon is sharply transected deep into the tendon sheath with the #15 blade releasing the tendon by cutting it into the medial wall of the calcaneus. A tendon passing suture technique with either absorbable or nonabsorbable suture is passed through the free end of the FHL tendon.

The authors' preferred method of transfer and fixation is through a calcaneal bone tunnel with interference screw fixation, as described by DeCarbo and Hyer.[64] A guide wire for the interference screw is placed in the posterior aspect of the calcaneus just anterior to Achilles tendon insertion point. The guide is angled slightly distal so the line of pull of the transferred tendon is not parallel to the vertical force of the Achilles tendon. The usual interference screw size is 7 mm × 23 mm. This interference screw size is the smallest diameter screw with the longest length. An overdrill creating the osseous bone tunnel is performed over the guide wire of 7 mm or 7.5 mm to ensure a tight secure fixation between the transferred tendon, interference screw, and osseous tunnel. The authors prefer the osseous tunnel to exit the plantar calcaneal

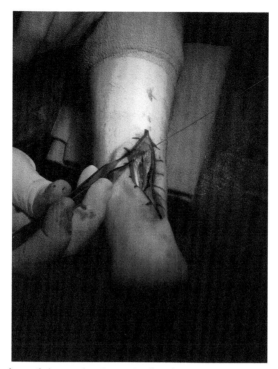

Fig. 7. Ventral surface of the tendon is repaired with 0 Vicryl in a running interlocking suture technique.

cortex; however, the tunnel only needs to be slightly deeper than the interference screw length (**Fig. 11**).

Once the tunnel is created, the suture through the FHL tendon is passed through the eye hole of the guide wire. The guide wire and the FHL tendon suture are pulled plantar exiting the foot. The suture is grabbed with a hemostat and the FHL tendon is guided into the osseous calcaneal tunnel while gently pulling the suture distally. The tension is set by pulling on the plantar suture through the skin. Maximal or near-maximal plantarflexion is desired due to the soft tissue stretching out over time. When the tension is set, an interference screw is placed into the osseous bone tunnel capturing the FHL tendon (**Fig. 12**).

Once stability is confirmed with gentle dorsiflexion of the ankle, the Achilles tendon that was previously débrided is repaired, as described previously. After the Achilles is repaired and the FHL tendon is transferred, the 2 tendons can be sutured together with a side-to-side anastomosis stitch. This allows the posterior compartment muscles to act as 1 unit to increase strength. Absorbable or nonabsorbable suture can be used and 0 grade is preferred. The incision is closed in layers, as described previously.

OUTCOMES

There is a wide variety of surgical procedures described for the treatment of midsubstance Achilles tendinopathy. Worse outcomes with surgical treatment have been reported in nonathletes.[67] Success rates between 75% and 100% have been reported with open procedures.[61,68–71] Recently, minimally invasive procedures were

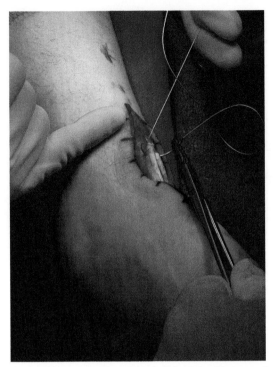

Fig. 8. Posterior surface of the tendon is repaired with 0 Vicryl in a running interlocking suture technique.

proposed. Paratenon or adhesion release, paratenon excision, ventral scraping, and tenotomies or microtenotomies with radiofrequency ablation have previously been described through open or minimally invasive approaches. For more advanced Achilles degeneration, excision of intratendinous lesions, FHL tendon transfers, or turndown flaps can supplement the procedure.

Systematic Reviews

Baltes and colleagues[72] in 2016 reported patient satisfaction for studies involving midsubstance Achilles tendinopathy. Studies reporting surgical management of noninsertional tendinopathy were included. If there was not a clear distinction between insertional and noninsertional Achilles tendinopathy the studies were excluded. Overall they noted low research methodology with heterogenous patient populations and heterogenous outcome measures with wide variations in results. For this reason they avoided data pooling and noted their conclusions require further substantiation. They did note worse results with isolated longitudinal tenotomies. They noted similar patient satisfaction with open versus minimally invasive procedures.

Lohrer and colleagues[73] in 2016 reported success rate and patient satisfaction for studies involving midsubstance Achilles tendinopathy. Insertional Achilles tendinopathy was listed as exclusion criteria but some studies in the FHL tendon transfer subgroup were included without a clear distinction if patients had insertional or noninsertional tendinopathy.[74,75] Additionally, 1 of the studies on gastrocnemius recession included insertional Achilles tendinopathy patient outcomes in the patient satisfaction score.[76] Despite these flaws in methodology, the remaining pooled data

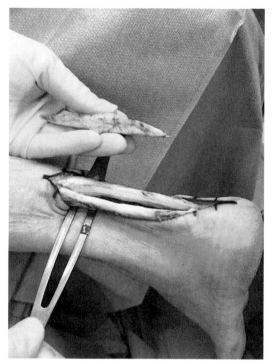

Fig. 9. Extensive degeneration with excision of greater than 50% of the Achilles tendon thickness.

for subgroups without intratendinous lesions offer the best available comparison of outcomes. The authors note open peritendinous débridement had statistically significant improved patient satisfaction compared with minimally invasive paratenon débridement, percutaneous longitudinal tenotomies, or open longitudinal tenotomies. Their conclusions require further evidence because they are based on a small number of studies that did not use validated outcome measures.

Paratenon Release and Excision of Intratendinous Lesion Results

Often studies report outcomes for paratenon release and excision of core tendinopathy lesions in the same case series. Three separate studies reported success rate for surgical treatment with and without a core area of tendinopathy. Lohrer and Nauck[77] performed a level 2 study with open release of the Achilles tendon and scarification for tendinopathy and open release with excision of intratendinous lesion when a central core lesion was appreciated on MRI. Nelen and colleagues[68] performed a level 4 study with open release of the Achilles tendon and excision of inflamed paratenon for paratendinopathy, open débridement was performed for tendinopathy. Paavola and colleagues[70] performed release of peritendinous adhesions for Achilles tendinopathy without a central core lesion and release of peritendinous adhesions with longitudinal excision of tendinopathy for Achilles tendinopathy with a core lesion.

The pooled data from 3 studies reveal a higher success rate with isolated paratenon release in the absence of a core area of Achilles tendinopathy (**Table 1**). Release of the paratenon in the absence of a core lesion had a success rate of 113 of 124 (91.1%). Success rate for longitudinal excision of a core lesion with side-to-side repair in these

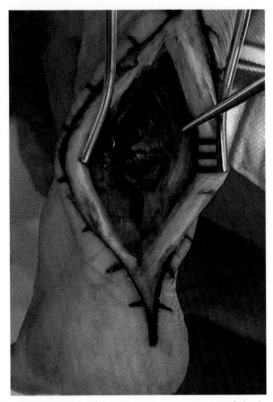

Fig. 10. FHL tendon is identified in the posterior compartment of the leg, where it courses between the posterior processes of the talus.

studies was 61 of 76 (80.3%). Patients without a core lesion who undergo release of the Achilles tendon may have better results compared with patients undergoing excision of tendinopathy.

Recently, Bedi and colleagues[78] found 14 of 15 high-level athletes had a successful result with ventral paratendinous scrapings and excision of adhered plantaris. Victorian Institute of Sports Assessment - Achilles Questionnaire (VISA-A) scores improved from 51 preoperatively to 95 postoperatively with improved tendon structure on postoperative ultrasound. This technique has shown promising results but requires further validation.

Flexor Hallucis Longus Tendon Transfer Results

Many outcome studies are available for FHL tendon transfer in the treatment of Achilles tendinopathy; however, only 1 FHL tendon outcome study is specific for noninsertional Achilles tendinopathy. Lui[79] presented the results of FHL tendon transfer with endoscopic débridement in 5 patients who had noninsertional Achilles tendinopathy. All patients had symptoms for at least 6 months' duration with at least 50% of the tendon involved on preoperative MRI. One patient had a poor functional result but had a severe crush injury to the affected extremity; the other 4 patients had excellent results. Martin and colleagues[80] reported on 56 patients who underwent complete excision of the Achilles tendon with FHL tendon transfer. Of the 44 patients available

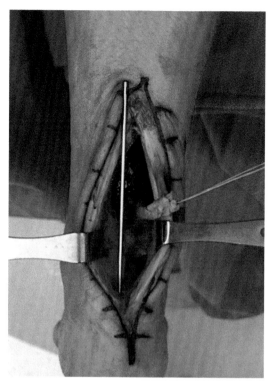

Fig. 11. FHL tendon resected with adequate length. Whipstitch has been performed through the FHL tendon with a tunnel created through the superior surface of the calcaneus.

for questionnaire 3.4 years postprocedure, 38 (86%) were satisfied with the procedure. Average American Orthopedic Foot and Ankle Score (AOFAS) for 19 patients available for objective assessment was 91.6. A turndown flap of the gastrocnemius aponeurosis is an alternative to FHL tendon transfers. Nelen and colleagues[68] noted improved patient satisfaction when a turndown flap supplemented débridement of extensive Achilles tendinopathy.

Gastrocnemius Recession Results

Strayer gastrocnemius recession has shown excellent results in recalcitrant noninsertional Achilles tendinopathy. Duthon and colleagues[81] reported an average postoperative AOFAS of 100 at 1-year follow-up in 14 patients; 8 of these patients who underwent postoperative MRI showed decreased intrasubstance signal intensity; 13 of 14 patients in the study were satisfied at 2-year follow-up.

Proximal medial gastrocnemius recession has shown better outcomes in noninsertional Achilles tendinopathy compared with insertional Achilles tendinopathy at 2.5-year follow-up.[76] All 5 patients who underwent gastrocnemius recession for noninsertional Achilles tendinopathy were highly satisfied, whereas only 2 of 5 patients who underwent gastrocnemius recession for insertional Achilles tendinopathy were satisfied with the procedure. For noninsertional Achilles tendinopathy, postoperative AOFAS was 91.2, postoperative VISA-A was 94, and postoperative visual analog scale was 0.4. For insertional Achilles tendinopathy, postoperative AOFAS was 78.2, postoperative VISA-A was 73.6, and postoperative visual analog scale was 5.6.

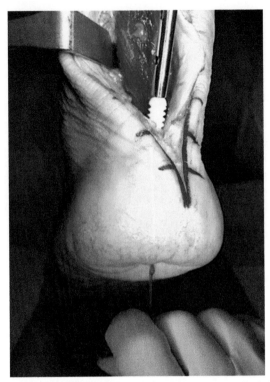

Fig. 12. The foot is held in plantarflexion and the FHL tendon is pulled through the tunnel with the desired tension. The interference screw is then inserted.

Noninsertional Achilles tendinopathy is commonly seen in athletes and despite encouraging results with gastrocnemius lengthening there is concern it may have a negative impact on athletic performance.[82] It is not known if excellent outcomes with gastrocnemius recession apply to patients with extensive degeneration.

The pathophysiology of noninsertional Achilles tendinopathy is poorly understood and there is a wide variety of surgical procedures. Three separate systematic reviews noted improved Coleman Methodology Scores with time, indicating higher-quality studies are being performed but there is still need for improvement.[61,72,73] RCTs are needed to compare surgical treatment to nonsurgical treatment in recalcitrant noninsertional Achilles tendinopathy. RCTs are needed to compare procedures that address Achilles paratendinopathy without a core area of tendinopathy, and separate

Table 1		
Success rates of paratenon release versus excision tendinopathy		
Authors	**Success Rates of Paratenon Release**	**Success Rates of Excision Tendinopathy**
Lohrer and Nauck,[77] 2014	15/15 (100%)	23/24 (95.8%)
Nelen et al,[68] 1989	82/93 (88.2%)	19/26 (73.1%)
Paavola et al,[70] 2002	16/16 (100%)	19/26 (73.1%)
Total	113/124 (91.1%)	61/76 (80.3%)

RCTs are needed to compare procedures that address the Achilles with a core area of tendinopathy. More outcome studies are needed that use validated outcome measures specific for Achilles tendinopathy, such as VISA-A.

COMPLICATIONS AND MANAGEMENT

Complications reported with open procedures for Achilles tendinopathy are not uncommon. Paavola and colleagues[83] have reported an overall complication rate of 11% in 432 patients with wound necrosis of 3%, superficial infection of 2.5%, and sural nerve injury of 1%. Seroma formation, hematoma formation, and hypertrophic scar formation each had an incidence of 1% and 1 patient in the series experienced a deep vein thrombosis. The total reoperation rate was 3%.

Two separate systematic reviews found a lower complication rate with minimally invasive procedures.[72,73] Lohrer and colleagues[73] reported a complication rate of 10.5% with open procedures compared with 5.3% in minimally invasive procedures. A higher complication rate is expected with open procedures due to poor vascularity in the area with a propensity for dehiscence. Because 1 of the main complications involves the soft tissue in this surgical area, special attention to retraction must be used to prevent pressure necrosis from aggressive tissue handling.

POSTOPERATIVE CARE

Postoperatively the initial protocol for midsubstance Achilles repair is placing the patient in a bulky jones compression dressing in gravity equinus for 7 to 10 days. At the first postoperative visit, the sutures are removed and the patient is placed into a slightly plantarflexed non–weight-bearing below-knee cast for 3 weeks. One month postoperatively, patients are transitioned out of the cast into a tall controlled ankle motion walking boot gradually progressing to a full weight-bearing boot with open kinetic chain range of motion. The boot walker is for an additional 3 weeks followed by an ankle brace with formal therapy for 1 month. Patients can come out of the ankle brace after 2 weeks in everyday life. At that point they are instructed to only wear the brace during periods of increased activity.

SUMMARY

In conclusion, midsubstance Achilles tendinopathy can be treated successfully in most instances with conservative care. If conservative care fails to provide pain relief or a functional return to activity, surgical intervention should be considered. Conservative treatment should be exhausted for 3 to 6 months before surgical treatment is offered unless there is extensive degeneration. When surgical débridement is considered, the authors prefer an open technique. This allows direct visualization and débridement of the diseased tendon with primary repair. This technique has low patient morbidity and low postoperative complications. When there is concern regarding the tensile strength of the repair, the authors prefer an FHL tendon transfer. Isolated open ventral paratenon release or scraping may be considered in athletes without a core area of tendinopathy on MRI.

REFERENCES

1. van Dijk CN, van Sterkenburg MN, Wiegerinck JI, et al. Terminology for Achilles tendon related disorders. Knee Surg Sports Traumatol Arthrosc 2011;19:835–41.
2. Maffulli N, Kader D. Tendinopathy of tendo Achillis. J Bone Joint Surg Br 2002;84: 1–8.

3. Åström M, Rausing A. Chronic Achilles tendinopathy. A survey of surgical and histopathologic findings. Clin Orthop 1995;316:151–64.

4. Kannus P, Niittymäki S, Järvinen M, et al. Sports injuries in elderly athletes: a three-year prospective, controlled study. Age Ageing 1989;18:263–70.

5. de Jonge S, van den Berg C, de Vos RJ, et al. Incidence of midportion Achilles tendinopathy in the general population. Br J Sports Med 2011;45:1026–8.

6. Lysholm J, Wiklander J. Injuries in runners. Am J Sports Med 1987;15:168–71.

7. Maffulli N, Khan KM, Puddu G. Overuse tendon conditions: time to change a confusing terminology. Arthroscopy 1998;14:840–3.

8. Perry JR. Achilles tendon anatomy: normal and pathologic. Foot Ankle Clin 1997; 2:363–70.

9. Kannus P. Structure of the tendon connective tissue. Scand J Med Sci Sports 2000;10:312–20.

10. Fratzl P. Cellulose and collagen: from fibrils to tissue. Curr Opin Colloid Interface Sci 2009;8:32–9.

11. Kirkendall DT, Garrett WE. Function and biomechanics of tendons. Scand J Med Sci Sports 1997;7:62–6.

12. Carr AJ, Norris SH. The blood supply of the calcaneal tendon. J Bone Joint Surg Br 1989;71:100–1.

13. Lagergren C, Lindholm A. Vascular distribution in the Achilles tendon; an angiographic and microangiographic study. Acta Chir Scand 1959;116:491–5.

14. Åström M, Westlin N. Blood flow in the human Achilles tendon assessed by laser doppler flowmetry. J Orthop Res 1994;12:246–52.

15. Stein V, Laprell H, Tinnemeyer S, et al. Quantitative assessment of intravascular volume of the human Achilles tendon. Acta Orthop Scand 2000;71:60–3.

16. Chen TM, Rozen WM, Pan WR, et al. The arterial anatomy of the Achilles tendon: anatomical study and clinical implications. Clin Anat 2009;22:377–85.

17. Schepsis AA, Jones H, Haas AL. Achilles tendon disorders in athletes. Am J Sports Med 2002;30:287–305.

18. Fredericson M. Common injuries in runners. Diagnosis, rehabilitation and prevention. Sports Med 1996;21:49–72.

19. DeMaio M, Paine K, Drez D. Achilles tendonitis. Orthopedics 1995;18:195–204.

20. Fornage BD. Achilles tendon: US examination. Radiology 1986;159:759–64.

21. Sandmeier R, Renström PA. Diagnosis and treatment of chronic tendon disorders in sports. Scand J Med Sci Sports 1997;7:96–106.

22. Paavola M, Kannus P, Järvinen TA, et al. Achilles tendinopathy. J Bone Joint Surg Am 2002;84A:2062–76.

23. Pope CF. Radiologic evaluation of tendon injuries. Clin Sports Med 1992;11: 579–99.

24. Järvinen TA, Kannus P, Paavola M, et al. Achilles tendon injuries. Curr Opin Rheumatol 2001;13:150–5.

25. Alfredson H, Ohberg L, Forsgren S. Is vasculo-neural ingrowth the cause of pain in chronic Achilles tendinosis? An investigation using ultrasonography and colour Doppler, immunohistochemistry, and diagnostic injections. Knee Surg Sports Traumatol Arthrosc 2003;11:334–8.

26. Schubert TE, Weidler C, Lerch K, et al. Achilles tendinosis is associated with sprouting of substance P positive nerve fibres. Ann Rheum Dis 2005;64:1083–6.

27. Lian Ø, Dahl J, Ackermann PW, et al. Pronociceptive and antinociceptive neuromediators in patellar tendinopathy. Am J Sports Med 2006;34:1801–8.

28. Tol JL, Spiezia F, Maffulli N. Neovascularization in Achilles tendinopathy: have we been chasing a red herring? Knee Surg Sports Traumatol Arthrosc 2012;20: 1891–4.

29. Sengkerij PM, de Vos RJ, Weir A, et al. Interobserver reliability of neovascularization score using power Doppler ultrasonography in midportion achilles tendinopathy. Am J Sports Med 2009;37:1627–31.

30. Richards PJ, McCall IW, Day C, et al. Longitudinal microvascularity in Achilles tendinopathy (power Doppler ultrasound, magnetic resonance imaging time-intensity curves and the Victorian Institute of Sport Assessment-Achilles questionnaire): a pilot study. Skeletal Radiol 2010;39:509–21.

31. De Jonge S, Warnaars JL, De Vos RJ, et al. Relationship between neovascularization and clinical severity in Achilles tendinopathy in 556 paired measurements. Scand J Med Sci Sports 2014;24:773–8.

32. Kannus P, Jozsa L. Histopathological changes preceding spontaneous rupture of a tendon: a controlled study of 891 patients. J Bone Joint Surg Am 1991;73: 1507–25.

33. Rolf C, Movin T. Etiology, histopathology, and outcome of surgery in achillodynia. Foot Ankle Int 1997;18:565–9.

34. Riley G. The pathogenesis of tendinopathy: a molecular perspective. Rheumatology 2004;43:131–42.

35. Fredberg U, Stengaard-Pedersen K. Chronic tendinopathy tissue pathology, pain mechanisms, and etiology with a special focus on inflammation. Scand J Med Sci Sports 2008;18:3–15.

36. Rees JD, Maffulli N, Cook J. Management of tendinopathy. Am J Sports Med 2009;37:1855–67.

37. Torp-Pedersen TE, Torp-Pedersen ST, Qvistgaard E, et al. Effect of gluco- corticosteroid injections in tennis elbow verified on colour Doppler ultrasonography: evidence of inflammation. Br J Sports Med 2008;42:978–82.

38. Hart L. Corticosteroid and other injections in the management of tendinopathies: a review. Clin J Sport Med 2011;21:540–1.

39. Shrier I, Matheson GO, Kohl HW. Achilles tendonitis: are corticosteroid injections useful or harmful? Clin J Sport Med 1996;6:245–50.

40. Mafi N, Lorentzon R, Alfredson H. Superior short-term results with eccentric calf muscle training compared to concentric training in a randomized prospective multicenter study on patients with chronic achilles tendinosis. Knee Surg Sports Traumatol Arthrosc 2001;9:42–7.

41. Stanish WD, Rubinovich RM, Curwin S. Eccentric exercise in chronic tendinitis. Clin Orthop Relat Res 1986;(208):65–8.

42. Magnussen RA, Dunn WR, Thomson AB. Nonoperative treatment of midportion Achilles tendinopathy: a systematic review. Clin J Sport Med 2009;19:54–64.

43. Rees JD, Lichtwark GA, Wolman RL, et al. The mechanism for efficacy of eccentric loading in Achilles tendon injury; an in vivo study in humans. Rheumatology 2008;47:1493–7.

44. Alfredson H, Pietilä T, Jonsson P, et al. Heavy-load eccentric calf muscle training for the treatment of chronic Achilles tendinosis. Am J Sports Med 1998;26:360–6.

45. Silbernagel KG, Thomee R, Eriksson BI, et al. Continued sports activity, using a pain-monitoring model, during rehabilitation in patients with Achilles tendinopathy: a randomized controlled study. Am J Sports Med 2007;35:897–906.

46. Roos EM, Engström M, Lagerquist A, et al. Clinical improvement after 6 weeks of eccentric exercise in patients with mid-portion achilles tendinopathy: a randomized trial with 1-year follow-up. Scand J Med Sci Sports 2004;14:286–95.

47. Verrall G, Schofield S, Brustad T. Chronic Achilles tendinopathy treated with eccentric stretching program. Foot Ankle Int 2011;32:843–9.
48. Meyer A, Tumilty S, Baxter GD. Eccentric exercise protocols for chronic non-insertional achilles tendinopathy: how much is enough? Scand J Med Sci Sports 2009;19:609–15.
49. Beyer R, Kongsgaard M, Hougs Kjær B, et al. Heavy slow resistance versus eccentric training as treatment for achilles tendinopathy: a randomized controlled trial. Am J Sports Med 2015 Jul;43:1704–11.
50. Rompe JD, Furia J, Maffulli N. Eccentric loading versus eccentric loading plus shock-wave treatment for midportion achilles tendinopathy: a randomized controlled trial. Am J Sports Med 2009;37:463–70.
51. Rasmussen S, Christensen M, Mathiesen I, et al. Shockwave therapy for chronic Achilles tendinopathy: a double-blind, randomized clinical trial of efficacy. Acta Orthop 2008;79:249–56.
52. de Jonge S, de Vos RJ, Weir A, et al. One-year follow-up of platelet-rich plasma treatment in chronic Achilles tendinopathy: a double-blind randomized placebo-con- trolled trial. Am J Sports Med 2011;39:1623–9.
53. de Mos M, van der Windt AE, Jahr H, et al. Can platelet-rich plasma enhance tendon repair? A cell culture study. Am J Sports Med 2008;36:1171–8.
54. Schnabel LV, Mohammed HO, Miller BJ, et al. Platelet rich plasma (PRP) en-hances anabolic gene expression patterns in flexor digitorum superficialis ten-dons. J Orthop Res 2007;25:230–40.
55. Klein MB, Yalamanchi N, Pham H, et al. Flexor tendon healing in vitro: effects of TGF-beta on tendon cell collagen production. J Hand Surg Am 2002;27:615–20.
56. De Vos RJ, Weir A, Tol JL, et al. No effects of PRP on ultrasonographic tendon structure and neovascularisation in chronic midportion Achilles tendinopathy. Br J Sports Med 2011;45:387–92.
57. de Vos RJ, Weir A, van Schie HT, et al. Platelet-rich plasma injection for chronic Achilles tendinopathy: a randomized controlled trial. JAMA 2010;303:144–9.
58. Sadoghi P, Rosso C, Valderrabano V, et al. The role of platelets in the treatment of achilles tendon injuries. J Orthop Res 2013;31:111–8.
59. Nicholson CW, Berlet GC, Lee TH. Prediction of the success of nonoperative treatment of insertional Achilles tendinosis based on MRI. Foot Ankle Int 2007; 28:472–7.
60. Nehrer S, Breitenseher M, Brodner W, et al. Clinical and sonographic evaluation of the risk of rupture in the Achilles tendon. Arch Orthop Trauma Surg 1997;116: 14–8.
61. Tallon C, Coleman BD, Khan KM, et al. Outcome of surgery for chronic Achilles tendinopathy: a critical review. Am J Sports Med 2001;29:315–20.
62. Attinger CE, Evans KK, Bulan E, et al. Angiosomes of the foot and ankle and clin-ical implications for limb salvage: reconstruction, incisions, and revascularization. Plast Reconstr Surg 2006;117:261S–93S.
63. Silver RL, de la Garza J, Rang M. The myth of muscle balance: a study of relative strengths and excursions of normal muscles about the foot and ankle. J Bone Joint Surg Br 1985;67:432–7.
64. DeCarbo WT, Hyer CF. Interference screw fixation for flexor hallucis longus tendon transfer for chronic Achilles tendonopathy. J Foot Ankle Surg 2008;47: 69–72.
65. White RK, Kraynick BM. Surgical uses of the peroneus brevis tendon. Surg Gyne-col Obstet 1959;108:117–21.

66. Nunley JA, Ruskin G, Horst F. Long-term clinical outcomes following the central incision technique for insertional Achilles tendinopathy. Foot Ankle Int 2011;32: 850–5.
67. Maffulli N, Testa V, Capasso G, et al. Surgery for chronic Achilles tendinopathy yields worse results in nonathletic patients. Clin J Sport Med 2006;16:123–8.
68. Nelen G, Martens M, Burssens A. Surgical treatment of chronic Achilles tendinitis. Am J Sports Med 1989;17:754–9.
69. Schepsis AA, Leach RE. Surgical management of Achilles tendinitis. Am J Sports Med 1987;15:308–15.
70. Paavola M, Kannus P, Orava S, et al. Surgical treatment for chronic Achilles tendinopathy: a prospective seven month follow up study. Br J Sports Med 2002;36: 178–82.
71. Maffulli N, Testa V, Capasso G, et al. Results of percutaneous longitudinal tenotomy for Achilles tendinopathy in middle and long-distance runners. Am J Sports Med 1997;25:835–40.
72. Baltes TP, Zwiers R, Wiegerinck JI, et al. Surgical treatment for midportion Achilles tendinopathy: a systematic review. Knee Surg Sports Traumatol Arthrosc 2016. http://dx.doi.org/10.1007/s00167-016-4062-9.
73. Lohrer H, David S, Nauck T. Surgical treatment for achilles tendinopathy - a systematic review. BMC Musculoskelet Disord 2016;17:207.
74. Wilcox DK, Bohay DR, Anderson JG. Treatment of chronic achilles tendon disorders with flexor hallucis longus tendon transfer/augmentation. Foot Ankle Int 2000;21:1004–10.
75. Cottom JM, Hyer CF, Berlet GC, et al. Flexor hallucis tendon transfer with an interference screw for chronic Achilles tendinosis: a report of 62 cases. Foot Ankle Spec 2008;1:280–7.
76. Gurdezi S, Kohls-Gatzoulis J, Solan MC. Results of proximal medial gastrocnemius release for Achilles tendinopathy. Foot Ankle Int 2013;34:1364–9.
77. Lohrer H, Nauck T. Results of operative treatment for recalcitrant retrocalcaneal bursitis and midportion Achilles tendinopathy in athletes. Arch Orthop Trauma Surg 2014;134:1073–81.
78. Bedi HS, Jowett C, Ristanis S, et al. Plantaris excision and ventral Paratendinous Scraping for Achilles Tendinopathy in an Athletic Population. Foot Ankle Int 2016; 37:386–93.
79. Lui TH. Treatment of chronic noninsertional Achilles tendinopathy with endoscopic Achilles tendon debridement and flexor hallucis longus transfer. Foot Ankle Spec 2012;5:195–200.
80. Martin RL, Manning CM, Carcia CR, et al. An outcome study of chronic Achilles tendinosis after excision of the Achilles tendon and flexor hallucis longus tendon transfer. Foot Ankle Int 2005;26:691–7.
81. Duthon VB, Lubbeke A, Duc SR, et al. Noninsertional Achilles tendinopathy treated with gastrocnemius lengthening. Foot Ankle Int 2011;32:375–9.
82. Nawoczenski DA, Barske H, Tome J, et al. Isolated gastrocnemius recession for achilles tendinopathy: strength and functional outcomes. J Bone Joint Surg Am 2015;97:99–105.
83. Paavola M, Orava S, Leppilahti J, et al. Chronic Achilles tendon overuse injury: complications after surgical treatment: an analysis of 432 consecutive patients. Am J Sports Med 2000;28:77–82.

Insertional Achilles Tendinopathy

Gage M. Caudell, DPM

KEYWORDS

- Achilles • Insertional Achilles • Achilles tendinopathy • Haglund deformity
- Retrocalcaneal exostosis

KEY POINTS

- Nonoperative treatment of insertional achilles tendinopathy has mixed evidence of success. There are many options but unfortunately many fail.
- Surgical management often times is successful in reducing patients discomfort and pain. There is no prospective studies that suggest one procedure over another.
- In the authors opinion, patients should be well educated on postoperative expectations and even though surgery is often successful, the recovery can take up to a year.

Posterior heel pain is a common entity, frequently involving the Achilles tendon. There are 2 categories of Achilles tendinopathy: insertional and noninsertional. Insertional Achilles tendinopathy accounts for 20% to 24% of all Achilles disorders.[1,2] There are a myriad of diagnoses that can present with symptoms reflective of insertional Achilles tendinopathy, such as Haglund deformity, retrocalcaneal bursitis, retrocalcaneal exostosis, and Achilles tendinosis. Most of these conditions often coexist and can confound the primary diagnosis of insertional Achilles tendinopathy. Noninsertional Achilles tendinopathy, which is not discussed in this article, is another common cause of Achilles tendon symptoms. It is important to distinguish between insertional and noninsertional Achilles tendinopathy because the treatment options differ.

First described by Patrick Haglund in 1928, the Haglund deformity is one of the primary causes of heel pain[3] (**Fig. 1**). Historically, it was defined as an enlarged posterosuperior border of the os calcis and was originally thought to be the result of wearing rigid, low-back shoes. Today it is defined by a combination of inflammation of the retrocalcaneal bursa and insertional Achilles tendinopathy. It is thought that the osseous

Disclosure: The author has no commercial or financial conflicts of interest or funding sources with regard to this article.
This article is modified and updated from an article written for The Podiatry Institute 2008 Update: Lin B, Caudell G, Krywiak A, Grossman J. Insertional Achilles tendinopathy. The Podiatry Institute 2008 Update, 2008;150–155.
Fort Wayne Orthopedics, 7601 West Jefferson Boulevard, Fort Wayne, IN 46804, USA
E-mail address: gage@caudell.me

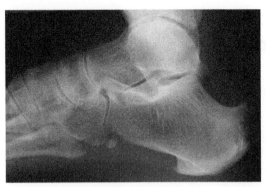

Fig. 1. Lateral weight-bearing radiograph showing Haglund deformity. Note the large eminence on the posterosuperior margin of the calcaneal tuberosity.

protuberance impinges on the retrocalcaneal bursa causing an inflammatory reaction.[4] One of the primary causes of a Haglund deformity is related to a high calcaneal inclination angle, thus it is commonly associated with a cavovarus foot type. Clinically, patients present with posterosuperior or posterosuperior-lateral heel prominence, local erythema, effusion, and pain on dorsiflexion secondary to tethering of the anterior aspect of the Achilles tendon against the bursal projection.[2]

Retrocalcaneal bursitis, another component of heel pain, is commonly associated with Haglund deformity and rarely exists independently of other coexisting conditions. The retrocalcaneal bursa is located just superior and anterior to the insertion of the Achilles tendon.[4] This condition can be unilateral or bilateral and is typically caused by shoe gear irritation in runners and in people who wear high-heeled shoes. The chief complaint is posterior heel pain, which typically worsens with activity.[3] Clinically, bursitis presents with pain to palpation anterior to both the medial and lateral margins of the Achilles tendon. This clinical finding distinguishes it from other types of posterior heel disorder.[2]

Retrocalcaneal exostosis is another common cause of posterior heel pain. It occurs mostly in middle-aged and elderly individuals, but can occur in younger individuals. The chief complaint and clinical findings are similar to those in Haglund deformity. There is often a palpable prominence in the Achilles tendon, most notably at its insertion. It is easy to differentiate from Haglund deformity by location. A true Haglund deformity is a posterosuperior or posterosuperior-lateral calcaneal prominence, whereas retrocalcaneal exostosis has an intratendinous component and is typically located 1 to 2 cm distal to the superior aspect of the posterior calcaneal tubercle[4,5] (**Fig. 2**). Unlike Haglund deformity, a retrocalcaneal exostosis does not have an association with a high inclination area.[6]

In addition, insertional Achilles tendinosis is a chronic condition often associated with overuse and chronic pull of the tendon on the posterior aspect of the heel. Tendinosis is seen typically in Haglund deformity at the anterior aspect of the tendon at the bursal projection. As the foot dorsiflexes during gait, the tendon glides against the posterosuperior prominence of the calcaneus causing pathologic changes within the tendon. Retrocalcaneal exostosis typically presents with thickening and calcific changes of the Achilles tendon at its insertion caused by repetitive pulling and microtearing. According to Paavola and colleagues,[7] these degenerative processes may be secondary to hypoxic degeneration, hyaline degeneration, mucoid or myxoid degeneration, fibrinoid degeneration, fatty degeneration, calcification, and fibrocartilaginous or osseous metaplasia.

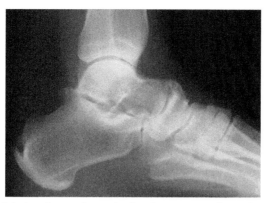

Fig. 2. Lateral weight-bearing radiograph showing a retrocalcaneal exostosis. Note the large spur and calcification at the insertion of the Achilles tendon.

The cause of insertional Achilles tendinopathy is multifactorial. It is typically broken down into intrinsic and extrinsic risk factors. Intrinsic risk factors include structural or biomechanical foot, ankle, and lower extremity conditions. Common extrinsic factors are overtraining, improper stretching/preparation, shoe gear, obesity, age, and mechanical overload.[8–11] All of these causes are anecdotal and have yet to be proved.

New evidence provided by Lyman and colleagues,[12] Rufai and colleagues,[13] and Benjamin and colleagues[5] in separate studies suggests that the calcification seen in these individuals is related to stress shielding forces. This adaptation increases the surface area at the bone-tendon junction, thereby protecting this area from increased mechanical loads.[5,12,13]

IMAGING

Three imaging modalities aid in the diagnosis of Achilles tendinopathy: plain radiographs, MRI, and ultrasonography. Plain radiographs are useful in the diagnosis of Haglund deformity, retrocalcaneal exostosis, and intratendinous calcification. As previously described, Haglund deformity is most appreciated on lateral radiographs, which show a large posterosuperior prominence (bursal projection). An associated high calcaneal inclination angle is also common. Other angles including Fowler-Philip angle, parallel pitch lines, and total angle of Ruch have been used to describe this deformity.[14,15] Retrocalcaneal exostosis is again best viewed on lateral radiographs. The prominence presents at the main insertion of the Achilles tendon with enlargement of the posterior calcaneal tubercle and intratendinous calcification.

MRI may be beneficial in diagnosing inflammatory changes in the posterior heel soft tissues (bursitis), tendon tears or rupture, degenerative tendon thickening (tendinosis), and calcification in cases in which the clinical findings and symptoms do not allow the clinician to make a definitive diagnosis. Most cases of insertional tendinopathy have a typical symptom presentation and clinical findings on examination. In most cases plain film radiography is adequate for diagnosis and the expense of advanced imaging is not needed for confirmation when following treatment progress. As with degeneration, increased signal intensity is visualized within the tendon on T2 and decreased intensity on T1 (**Fig. 3**). The authors typically order MRI for surgical planning if there is concern about significant insertional Achilles tendinosis and possible need for complicated reconstruction and consideration for using flexor hallucis longus tendon transfer.

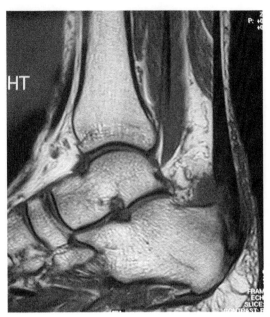

Fig. 3. Sagittal plain T1-weighted MRI shows a large Haglund deformity with associated Achilles tendon thickening and calcification.

Ultrasonography is beneficial in dynamic assessment of tendinopathy. It is also a fast and repeatable modality; however, it is very technician dependent. In a study reviewing histologic biopsy of injured Achilles and comparing it with the diagnosis made with modalities such as MRI or ultrasonography, MRI and ultrasonography provided similar findings.[16]

CONSERVATIVE TREATMENT

Initial treatment of any Achilles tendinopathy begins with RICE (rest, immobilization, compression, and elevation). The use of nonsteroidal antiinflammatory drugs (NSAIDs) has been advocated for Achilles tendinosis, but this practice is debatable. A study of the NSAID medication piroxicam found no benefit in treatment of Achilles tendinopathy.[17] Although NSAIDs may be helpful for pain modulation they do not treat the histologic abnormality of the tendon, which is degenerative and not inflammatory. Accommodative therapies, such as change of shoe gear (lower or no heel counter), addition of heel lifts, and orthotics, have shown relief of symptoms by relieving some of the mechanical stresses on the tissues, but these measures do not correct the underlying degenerative disorder. Some forms of physical therapy have shown success in symptom modulation and in some cases healing of the degenerative process, but rehabilitation programs do not show as high a success rate for insertional tendinopathy as for noninsertional tendinopathy. Gastrocnemius-soleus stretching exercises have shown improvement in symptoms in patients with retrocalcaneal exostosis and especially when there is coexisting equinus. Eccentric muscle strength training has been shown to reduce tendon thickening and decrease tendon neovascularization in noninsertional Achilles tendinopathy.[18] However, standard eccentric calf muscle training has not shown the same efficacy in insertional Achilles tendinopathy.

Fahlstrom and colleagues[19] found only 32% of patients with insertional Achilles tendinopathy to have improvement of symptoms when using eccentric strength training. Jonsson and colleagues[20] performed a pilot study of a modified eccentric calf muscle training regimen for patients with chronic insertional Achilles tendinopathy. This study of 27 patients with a total of 34 painful Achilles tendons had a success rate of 67%. Patients performed an eccentric training regimen without loading into dorsiflexion. This was accomplished by having patients perform a heel raise with the noninjured leg, then all body weight was transferred to the injured side and from the heel-raised position the patients slowly lowered the heel to floor level. This movement was done 3 times for 15 repetitions, twice a day, 7 d/wk for 12 weeks. If they had bilateral symptoms the patients performed a leg press while standing on a box or a staircase to avoid as much concentric load as possible.[20]

Therapeutic ultrasonography has also been used to increase the rate of collagen synthesis by providing silent mechanical vibration at high frequencies that penetrate the deep tissue. This modality may provide some symptomatic relief. The use of iontophoresis therapy, or the addition of topical steroids during ultrasonography treatment of heel pain, has been shown to provide some degree of symptomatic relief, although there are no studies showing its long-term efficacy. Extracorporeal shock wave therapy (ESWT) has been suggested to be effective in treating the symptoms of many chronic musculoskeletal conditions. A few small studies have investigated the use of ESWT in insertional Achilles tendinopathy.[21–23] Results so far seem to be promising but more research is needed.

The use of corticosteroid injections has been long debated with regard to tendon injection and most clinicians recommend that steroid injections into tendons should be used with caution because of the risk for potential tendon rupture. Low-dose injections of steroids into the retrocalcaneal bursa have not been shown to be dangerous and can provide some level of symptomatic relief. With regard to tendinopathy, the steroid does not alter the disease process because tendinopathy is largely degenerative and not inflammatory. Injections of many other substances have been used for tendon injection with good safety and clinical improvement. Even dry needling has shown favorable results, raising an interesting question of whether it is the insult of the needle stimulating a healing biological response or whether it is the pharmaceutical substance that provides the relief.

Prolotherapy has recently gained more acceptance in the musculoskeletal community because of its low cost and efficacy in the treatment of a variety of musculoskeletal problems. Prolotherapy is the injection or stimulation through mechanical insult to the tissue of growth factors to promote tissue repair or growth. This technique causes a brief inflammatory response in the stimulated tissue with a resultant release of cytokines and increase of growth factor activity, including chondrocytes, osteocytes, and fibroblasts. These growth factors help in resolving the musculoskeletal condition by allowing additional tissue growth and healing of the diseased tissue. There have been a few studies of the use of dextrose in the treatment of chronic Achilles tendinosis in both midportion and insertional Achilles tendinosis. None of these studies have shown the increased risk of tendon tear that is seen with corticosteroid injections.[24,25] Two prospective studies of both midportion Achilles and insertional Achilles tendinosis showed significant improvements. Yelland and colleagues[25] whet a step further by performing a randomized trial in which one group underwent prolotherapy injection and a second group underwent prolotherapy injection and eccentric loading exercises. The group that underwent both prolotherapy treatment with dextrose and eccentric loading exercises showed more rapid symptom relief.[24]

SURGICAL MANAGEMENT OF POSTERIOR HEEL DISORDER

There have been multiple procedures and techniques described for the surgical management of posterior heel disorder. Direct access to the pathologic posterior heel soft tissues can be obtained through more traditional open incisional endoscopic decompression, which has been purported to be effective in treating Haglund deformity and retrocalcaneal bursitis and to result in a better cosmetic appearance.[26] A variety of incisional approaches to access the posterior calcaneal soft tissues have been described, including, but not limited to, direct posterior central, lateral peritendinous, J shape, and transverse. The author typically approaches a Haglund deformity from a lateral approach unless there is significant calcific tendinosis and/or concurrent enthesophyte. The patient is placed in a lateral decubitus position or sometimes a supine position with a large bump when other procedures are to be performed. A thigh or calf tourniquet is used to facilitate hemostasis. The incision is made along the lateral wall of the calcaneal tubercle, just anterior to the anterior margin of the Achilles tendon (**Fig. 4**). The incision starts 2 cm proximal to the superior margin of the calcaneal tubercle and extends distally to the junction of the lateral and plantar skin. The incision is posterior to the course of the sural nerve, therefore it is made full thickness down to the calcaneal periosteum. Next, the retrocalcaneal bursa is typically observed and removed from the surgical site. Minimal lateral periosteal elevation is necessary to identify the posterosuperior calcaneal prominence. A retractor is placed into the wound and the Achilles is retracted posteriorly. An osteotome or sagittal saw is then used to remove the Haglund deformity. After removal of the prominence this is visualized under fluoroscopy so that adequate removal is noted. Next, the Achilles tendon is examined for any thickening or calcinosis. If significant disorder is identified, it is excised with care being taken not to debulk too much of the tendon. If only thickness is identified without calcification, radiofrequency ablation may be used. The wound is then flushed and, if significant periosteal elevation was necessary, suture anchors may be warranted. The author typically reapproximates the periosteum with absorbable sutures. The wound is then closed in layers. The author typically uses an absorbable suture for skin closure and applies 1.3-cm (0.5-inch) Steri-Strips. Nonadherent dressing is applied along with a 2-layer compression dressing and a posterior splint.

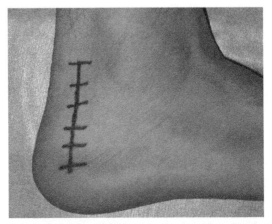

Fig. 4. Lateral incisional approach for removal of a Haglund deformity. The incision is extended proximal enough so excellent visualization can be obtained to successfully excise the posterosuperior prominence.

Retrocalcaneal exostosis is approached from a central posterior incision, beginning 2 cm proximal to the superior aspect of the calcaneus and extending 1 to 2 cm distal to the junction of the posterior and plantar skin (**Fig. 5**). The incision is made full thickness down to the deep fascia. Undermining is performed both medially and laterally releasing the subcutaneous tissue from the deep fascia. Next, a linear deep fascia and paratenon incision is performed midline from proximal to distal. The incision can be deepened full thickness through the Achilles tendon at its attachment to the calcaneus. The deep fascia and paratenon are then bluntly dissected as 1 unit from its attachment to the Achilles tendon. Even though at this level the Achilles does not glide extensively through the paratenon, reapproximation is important because it contributes to the blood supply of the tendon. The Achilles tendon is then sharply freed medially and laterally from its attachment to the calcaneal tuberosity with care taken to keep the most medial and lateral expansions of the tendon intact. At this time, direct visualization of the retrocalcaneal exostosis is accomplished (**Fig. 6**). A sagittal saw is used to remove the posterior prominence. If a Haglund deformity is present it is also excised at this time. Fluoroscopy is used to make sure all prominences are successfully removed. A reciprocating rasp is used to further contour the posterior calcaneal tuberosity and to roughen this area so that reattachment of the Achilles tendon can be facilitated. The wound is flushed and reattachment of the Achilles is initiated. There are a variety of ways to reapproximate the Achilles using such devices as screws, specialized plates or washers, and bone anchors. The use of posterior plating and tendon

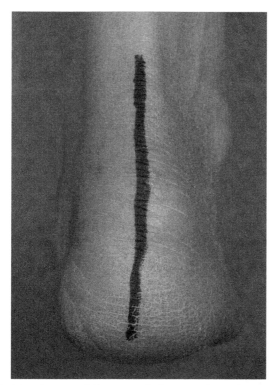

Fig. 5. Posterior incisional approach for removal of a retrocalcaneal exostosis. The incision is carried inferior so that visualization of the retrocalcaneal exostosis can be obtained and for the ability to easily reapproximate the Achilles tendon.

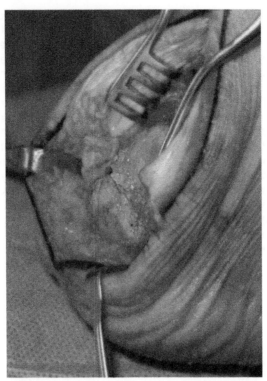

Fig. 6. Retrocalcaneal exostosis. As shown here, significant detachment of the Achilles tendon is needed for adequate visualization and removal of the spur.

washers carries the risk of posterior prominence and the need for removal, and has become less popular. More recently, knotless anchor systems have gained popularity. The author currently uses 4 anchors to reattach the Achilles to the posterior heel (**Fig. 7**). The construct consists of 2 anchors placed 1 cm proximal to the distal insertion of the Achilles tendon and central to each half of the tendon. Each anchor is double-loaded with strong nonabsorbable sutures that are color coded. One of the sutures is removed from each of the anchors, leaving one anchor with one color and the other with the other color. Next a single stitch is performed in each medial and lateral aspect of the Achilles tendon. Just distal to the end of the Achilles tendon insertion and directly inferior to the first row of anchor placements, a second row of anchors is created with a drill. One suture from each of the proximal anchors is passed through the eyelet of the anchor. Suture tension is achieved by pulling 1 suture at a time. With appropriate tension maintained on the sutures, the anchor is driven into the bone using a mallet. This process is then repeated to the fourth and final anchor. The ends of the suture are then cut as close to the cortex as possible. The resulting suture pattern should look similar to a capital M. The wound is then flushed and the deep fascia and paratenon are closed as 1 layer, followed by the subcutaneous layer and skin using an absorbable suture. Surgical glue is then also applied over the incision site. A 1-layer compression dressing is applied along with a posterior splint.

Postoperatively patients are non–weight bearing in a 2-layer compression dressing and posterior splint for 2 weeks until the incision is healed and, if nonabsorbable

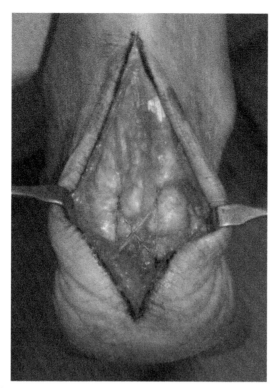

Fig. 7. The 4-anchor knotless anchor system. The suture bridge creates a figure-of-eight or M pattern. The implant is knotless, thus preventing any extra bulk to the posterior heel.

sutures are used, they are removed at this time. The patient is then placed in a compression stocking and removable boot for 4 weeks. If minimal detachment of the Achilles was performed, the patient may begin weight bearing in a cam boot at 2 weeks and resume using regular shoes at 4 weeks postoperatively. If significant detachment is performed, the patient is allowed protective weight bearing in a walker boot for a combined 6 weeks so that proper tendon healing can take place. At 6 weeks, the patient is allowed to return to regular shoes. Patients are encouraged not to return to any high-impact aerobic activity for at least 4 to 5 months postoperatively.

The most common complications in posterior heel surgery are wound healing complications.[27–29] The vascular supply to the posterior heel is often more delicate than in other parts of the foot and inherently creates the risk of delayed healing. Local wound care and antibiotics, if needed, assist in healing. If significant necrosis or exposed tendon occur, aggressive wound debridement may be necessary. Other complications include inadequate resection of bone, tendon rupture, and nerve entrapment.[27–29] The author has not encountered any tendon ruptures but has seen a few symptomatic nerve entrapments of branches of the lateral calcaneal nerve. In each case, sclerosing alcohol injections were used and uneventful resolution of symptoms occurred.

SUMMARY

In summary, insertional Achilles tendinopathy is associated with multiple causes and these are still debatable. After failing conservative treatment, surgical options are explored. This article focuses on 1 particular surgical technique, but there are many other ways to treat the pain of insertional Achilles tendinopathy. Regardless of the technique used, the goal of the procedure is to provide relief to the patient by removal of the calcaneal prominence and/or retrocalcaneal bursa.

REFERENCES

1. Astrom M, Rausing A. Chronic Achilles tendinopathy: a survey of surgical and histopathologic findings. Clin Orthop Relat Res 1995;(316):151–64.
2. Myerson M, McGarvey W. Disorders of the Achilles tendon insertion and Achilles tendinitis. Instr Course Lect 1999;48:211–8.
3. Watson A, Anderson R, Davis W. Comparison of results of retrocalcaneal decompression for retrocalcaneal bursitis and insertional Achilles tendinosis with calcific spur. Foot Ankle Int 2000;21(8):638–42.
4. McBryde A, Ortmann F. Retrocalcaneal buroscopy. Tech Foot Ankle Surg 2005; 4(3):174–9.
5. Benjamin M, Ruffian A, Ralphs J. The mechanism of formation of bony spurs (enthesophytes) in the Achilles tendon. Arthritis Rheum 2000;43(3):576–83.
6. Shibuya S, Thorud J, Agarwal M, et al. Is calcaneal inclination higher in patients with insertional Achilles tendinosis? A case controlled, cross-sectional study. J Foot Ankle Surg 2012;51:757–61.
7. Paavola M, Kannus P, Jarvinen T, et al. Achilles tendinopathy. J Bone Joint Surg Am 2002;84-A(11):2062–76.
8. Clement D, Taunton J, Smart G. Achilles tendinitis and peritendinitis: etiology and treatment. Am J Sports Med 1984;12:179–84.
9. Kaufman K, Brodine S, Shaffer R, et al. The effect of foot structure and range of motion on musculoskeletal overuse injuries. Am J Sports Med 1999;27(5):585–93.
10. Kvist M. Achilles tendon injuries in athletes. Ann Chir Gynaecol 1991;80:188–201.
11. Paavola M, Orava S, Leppilahti J, et al. Chronic Achilles tendon overuse injury: complications after surgical treatment. Am J Sports Med 2000;28(1):77–82.
12. Lyman J, Weinhold PS, Almekinders LC. Strain behavior of the distal Achilles tendon: implications for insertional Achilles tendinopathy. Am J Sports Med 2004;32:457–61.
13. Rufai A, Ralphs JR, Benjamin M. Structure and histopathology of the insertional region of the human Achilles tendon. J Orthop Res 1995;13:585–93.
14. Fowler A, Philip JF. Abnormality of the calcaneus as a cause of painful heel. Br J Surg 1954;32:494–500.
15. Heneghan MA, Pavlov H. The Haglund painful heel syndrome: experimental investigation of cause and therapeutic implications. Clin Orthop 1984;187: 228–34.
16. Astrom M, Gentz CF, Nilsson P, et al. Imaging in chronic Achilles tendinopathy: a comparison of ultrasonography, magnetic resonance imaging, and surgical findings in 27 histologically verified cases. Skeletal Radiol 1996;25:615–20.
17. Astrom M, Westlin N. No effect of piroxicam on Achilles tendinopathy: a randomized study of 70 patients. Acta Orthop Scand 1992;63:631–4.
18. Alfredson H, Pietila T, Jonsson P, et al. Heavy-load eccentric calf muscle training for the treatment of chronic Achilles tendinosis. Am J Sports Med 1998;26:360–6.
19. Fahlstrom M, Jonsson P, Lorentzon R, et al. Chronic Achilles tendon pain treated with eccentric calf muscle training. Knee Surg Sports Traumatol Arthrosc 2003; 11(5):327–33.

20. Jonsson P, Alfredson H, Sunding K, et al. New regimen for eccentric calf-muscle training in patients with chronic insertional Achilles tendinopathy: results of a pilot study. Br J Sports Med 2008;42:746–9.
21. Furia J. High-energy extracorporeal shock wave therapy as a treatment for insertional Achilles tendinopathy. Am J Sports Med 2006;34(5):733–40.
22. Furia J, Rompe J. Extracorporeal shock wave therapy in the treatment of chronic fasciitis and Achilles tendinopathy. Curr Opin Orthop 2007;18:102–11.
23. Rees J, Wilson A, Wolman R. Current concepts in the management of tendon disorders. Rheumatology (Oxford) 2006;45:508–21.
24. Ryan M, Wong A, Taunton J. Favorable outcome after sonographically guided intratendinous injection of hyperosmolar dextrose for chronic insertional and midportion Achilles tendinosis. AJR Am J Roentgenol 2010;194:1047–53.
25. Yelland M, Sweeting K, Lyftogt J, et al. Prolotherapy injections and eccentric loading exercises for painful Achilles tendinosis: a randomized trial. Br J Sports Med 2011;45:421–8.
26. Maffulli N, Testa V, Capasso G, et al. Calcific insertional Achilles tendinopathy: reattachment with bone anchors. Am J Sports Med 2004;32(1):174–82.
27. Gould J. Insertional tendinitis of the tendo Achilles. Tech Foot Ankle Surg 2005; 4(4):222–9.
28. Wagner E, Gould J, Kneidel M, et al. Technique and results of Achilles tendon detachment and reconstruction for insertional Achilles tendinosis. Foot Ankle Int 2006;27(9):677–84.
29. Aronow MS. Posterior heel pain (retrocalcaneal bursitis, insertional and noninsertional Achilles tendinopathy). Clin Podiatr Med Surg 2005;22:19–43.

Equinus and Lengthening Techniques

Patrick A. DeHeer, DPM[a,b,c],*

KEYWORDS

- Equinus • Achilles • Gastrocsoleal complex • Stretching • Bracing
- Tendo-Achilles lengthening • Strayer • Baumann

KEY POINTS

- Equinus is associated with the most biomechanically related lower extremity disorders.
- Global treatment of any disorder, either nonsurgical or surgical, requires treatment of any associated equinus.
- Tendo-Achilles lengthening is associated with higher complication rates, increased weakness, and prolonged healing compared with gastrocnemius recession (GR).
- GR is the procedure of choice for several recalcitrant lower extremity disorders (ie, plantar fasciitis, Achilles tendonitis/tendinosis, metatarsalgia, arch pain).
- The Baumann GR provides complete deformity correction with lower complication rates and less weakness compared with the Strayer GR.

INTRODUCTION

Equinus is associated in the literature with more than 30 lower extremity disorders, described as "the worst foot in the world is the one with a fully compensated equinus deformity," "the most profound causal agent in foot pathomechanics," and "the primary causal agent in a significant proportion of foot path ology"[1–40,41–69,70–89,80–118,119–141] (**Table 1**). Hill[1] found the incidence of equinus to be 96.5% for patients with a foot or ankle disorder. The importance of equinus was aptly described by Amis[12] in his outstanding article on equinus:

> It has been postulated that epidemiologic factors, such as obesity, sedentary life style, medical comorbidities, shoe wear, concrete floors, advanced age, female gender, and overuse issues, to name a few, are responsible for a variety of foot and ankle pathology. Although these factors might consistently coexist with a

Disclosure: The author is an owner of IQ Med and the inventor of The Equinus Brace.
[a] Surgery Department, Indiana University Health North Hospital, Carmel, IN, USA; [b] Surgery Department, Johnson Memorial Hospital, Franklin, IN, USA; [c] Department of Podiatric Medicine and Radiology, Rosalind Franklin University of Medicine and Science, North Chicago, IL, USA
* Corresponding author. 1159 West Jefferson Street, Suite 204, Franklin, IN 46131.
E-mail address: padeheer@sbcglobal.net

Table 1
Lower extremity disorders associated with equinus in the literature

Lower Extremity Orthopedic Disorder Related to Equinus	References
Plantar heel pain/plantar fasciitis	1,2,5–10,58–64,66,68–75,77,78,87,100–102,109,124–126,134
Achilles tendonitis/tendinosis	1,11–13,21,22,57,76,77,127–129,134,136,138–140
Posterior tibial tendon dysfunction/adult flat foot deformity	2,10,14–20,35,36,57,77,78,126,134,137,141
Muscle strains	23
Stress fractures	22,24,48,87
Shin splints/medial tibial stress syndrome	22,24,25,46,87
Iliotibial band syndrome	24,25
Patellofemoral syndrome	26,87
Ankle sprains/fractures	27
Diabetic foot ulcers	28–32,39,43,77,78,120–122,130–134
Charcot deformity	33,34,37–39
Metatarsalgia	1,2,6,10,16,20,36,41,77,124–126,134,135
MPJ synovitis/PDS	10
Hallux abductovalgus	1,2,16,20,40,52,65,77,126
Hammer toes/claw toes	20,44,77
Lisfranc/midfoot arthrosis	35,53,77,134
Hallux limitus/hallux rigidus	20,67
Forefoot calluses	1,20
Morton neuroma	38,45,77
Chronic ankle instability	47,87
Poor balance/increased fall rate in elderly	49,88
Sever disease	50,51
Pediatric flatfoot	54,55,137,141
Lateral foot pain	1
Genu recurvatum	38,41
Low back pain	38,41
Arch pain	6
Ankle arthrosis	77,78
Subtalar arthrosis	77
Sesamoiditis	77
Anterior compartment syndrome	87
Forefoot nerve entrapment	123

Abbreviations: MPJ, metatarsophalangeal joint; PDS, predislocation syndrome.

variety of foot and ankle problems and seem to have a causal relationship, it is my assertion that they have little if any direct relationship.

The singular and real association of each of these epidemiologic factors is a contracture of the gastrocnemius muscle, which is camouflaged in this list. Most every other cause of these foot and ankle problems is likely mediated by contributing to the degree and/or rate of an already contracting gastrocnemius.

These problems promote gastrocnemius tightness, which in time causes incremental damage to the foot and/or ankle.

Proper evaluation of equinus and an evidence-based definition are essential preliminary discussion points. Barouk and Barouk[41] described the proper technique as using the Silfverskiöld maneuver to differentiate gastrocnemius equinus (GE) from gastrocnemius-soleus equinus (GSE). The investigators stressed the importance of consistent examination methods during the examination, such as the amount of dorsiflexion pressure applied to the ball of the foot (moderate pressure consisting of <2 kg of applied force) and positioning of the hindfoot in either a neutral or a supinated position.[41] A goniometer is recommended by several investigators because of its ease of use and availability, despite poor reducibility[1–4,84,142–144] (**Figs. 1–6**).

The lack of a consistent definition for equinus has led to underdiagnosis and resultant undertreatment of equinus deformity. An evidence-based definition for equinus establishes consistency between researchers and clinicians for researching, evaluating, and treating equinus deformity. DiGiovanni and colleagues[2] offered an evidence-based definition for equinus. The recommended definition based on their study is ankle joint dorsiflexion of less than 5° with the knee extended for GE, and less than 10° with knee flexed for GSE[2] (**Table 2**).

The biomechanics of equinus explain the destructive consequences of a tight gastrocnemius-soleus complex (GSC). The GSC is the most significant medial arch flattening structure of the lower extremity.[145] Distal compensation results when a tight GSC does not allow the required 8° to 10° of ankle joint dorsiflexion for normal anterior advancement of the tibia over the foot during midstance, as well as proximal compensation occurring at the knee, hip, and lower back.[8,112,114] Specifically, increased tightness of the GSC results in a dampening of the frontal plane eversion of the medial column of the foot by the peroneus longus tendon resulting in dorsiflexion of the first metatarsal and cuneiform, and plantarflexion of the navicular and talus.[116] This lowering of the dome caused by equinus has been described in the literature for more than 100 years.[146]

INDICATIONS/CONTRAINDICATIONS

The indications for surgical lengthening of GE or GSE are self-evident: an equinus deformity that is present with or without an associated lower extremity disorder that

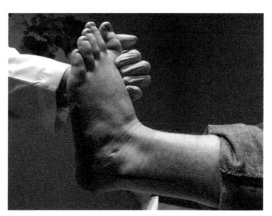

Fig. 1. Correct sagittal plane positioning of the foot in supination to evaluate ankle joint dorsiflexion locking the midtarsal joints and neutralizing the hindfoot position.

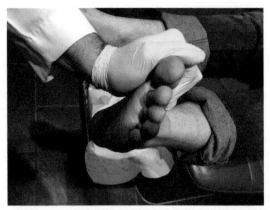

Fig. 2. Correct frontal plane positioning of the foot in supination to evaluate ankle joint dorsiflexion locking the midtarsal joints and neutralizing the hindfoot position.

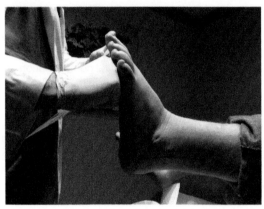

Fig. 3. Incorrect sagittal plane position of the foot in pronation to evaluate ankle joint dorsiflexion unlocking the midtarsal joints and pronating the hindfoot position, allowing dorsiflexion to occur in the midfoot.

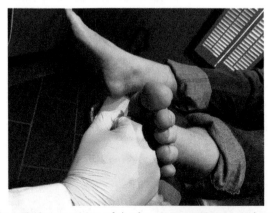

Fig. 4. Incorrect frontal plane position of the foot in pronation to evaluate ankle joint dorsiflexion unlocking the midtarsal joints and pronating the hindfoot position, allowing dorsiflexion to occur in the midfoot.

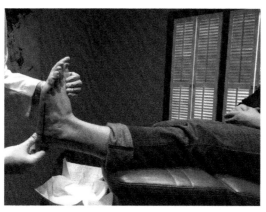

Fig. 5. Ankle joint dorsiflexion with the knee fully extended, evaluating for GE.

has not responded to conservative care. The salient point regarding indications is which GSC-lengthening surgical procedure is optimal. The initial decision point is tendo-Achilles lengthening (TAL) versus gastrocnemius recession (GR). The literature provides a clear answer. The Hoke triple hemisection was examined for accuracy of incision placement by Salomon and colleagues[147] in 2006. Correct incision placement was shown to range from 50% to 61% for each of the 3 incisions of the Hoke procedure.[147] In addition, several vital structures were shown to be within 1 cm of the incisions.[147] The complications associated with TAL are significant, especially overcorrection resulting in a calcaneal gait. The literature best shows calcaneal gait development in studies on diabetic forefoot ulcers treated with TAL resulting in plantar heel ulcers (**Table 3**). These high rates of heel ulceration rates associated with Achilles tendon insufficiency clearly shift the risk/benefit analysis toward GR.

The second decision point is which type of GR is preferred. The 2 main choices are the Strayer and Baumann procedures, with the primary differentiating factor being weakness. The Strayer procedure has a longer history and is more frequently used. The Strayer consists of a GR at the level of the gastrocnemius aponeurosis level.

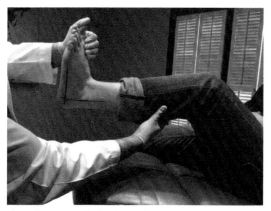

Fig. 6. Ankle joint dorsiflexion with the knee flexed, evaluating for gastrocnemius-soleus equinus.

Table 2 Definition of equinus deformities	
Ankle joint DF with KE <5°	GE
Ankle joint DF with KF <10°	Gastrocnemius-soleus equinus

Abbreviations: DF, dorsiflexion; GE, gastrocnemius equinus; KE, knee extended; KF, knee flexed.

The Strayer yields excellent correction of deformity but comes with a cost.[138,150] Molund and colleagues,[150] in their study of the Strayer procedure for multiple foot disorders, demonstrated a 22% reported plantarflexion weakness postoperatively. Nawoczenski and colleagues[138] concluded that, "Activities reported to be most problematic for GR participants (from the FAAM) included difficulty with ascending stairs/hills, running, jumping, cutting, and starting/stopping quickly. For patients who would like to participate in low to moderate levels of sports or activity, these deficits may not be relevant. However, an isolated GR may not be ideal for higher-level athletes who desire to participate in activities that require greater power production for performance."

The Baumann procedure is an intramuscular facial lengthening initially described 1989, and subsequently in English in 1992 as multiple gastrocnemius recessions.[151,152] The anatomic nomenclature is critical in differentiating the Strayer GR (aponeurotic lengthening) from the Baumann GR (fascial lengthening). The Baumann GR produces excellent deformity correction without weakness and overcorrection.[137,153–155]

SURGICAL TECHNIQUE/PROCEDURE
Preoperative Planning

Preoperative planning is fairly straightforward for equinus, especially with the Baumann GR, because it provides the ability to correct both GE and GSE deformities. The important principle is that, if the patient has an equinus deformity with an associated lower extremity, comprehensive surgical correction must include treatment of the equinus deformity.

Prep and Patient Positioning

One of the major advantages for the Baumann GR is that no special positioning of the patient is required. The procedure is performed with the patient in the supine position with standard prepping and draping to above the knee. Typically, a thigh tourniquet is used.

Surgical Approach

The surgical approach consists of a medial calf incision placed approximately 2 finger breadths below the anterior border of the tibia, just above the myotendinous junction. The incision is usually 4 to 6 cm in length and parallel to the anterior border of the tibia (**Fig. 7**).

Table 3 Heel ulceration rates after tendo-Achilles lengthening for forefoot ulcers	
Study	**Heel Ulceration Rate (%)**
Holstein et al,[148] 2004	16
Mueller et al,[31] 2003	13
Nishimoto et al,[32] 2003	2–10
Chilvers et al,[149] 2007	22

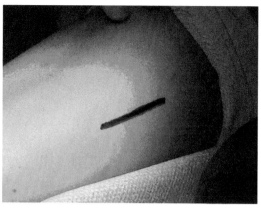

Fig. 7. Incision for Baumann GR located along the medial calf approximately 2 fingers below the anterior border of the tibia and just above the myotendinous junction, 4 to 6 cm in length.

Surgical Procedure

Step 1. The incision is made using a number 10 blade approximately 4 to 6 cm in length just through the skin (**Fig. 8**).

Step 2. Deepen the incision with Metzenbaum scissors to the level of deep fascia. If the great saphenous vein or saphenous nerve are encountered, they should be retracted anteriorly (**Fig. 9**).

Step 3. Digital blunt dissection helps to expose the deep fascial layer (**Fig. 10**).

Step 4. A self-retaining retractor such as a Weitlaner or Chung retractor is then inserted, exposing the deep fascial layer (**Figs. 11** and **12**).

Step 5. A hemostat is used to elevate the deep fascia, allowing incision via Metzenbaum scissors. Typically, the soleus muscle protrudes after incision of the deep fascia (**Fig. 13**).

Step 6. Use an index finger to identify the intramuscular interval between the gastrocnemius and soleus muscles. It is critical to avoid creating a false plane within one of the muscles by using excessive force (**Fig. 14**).

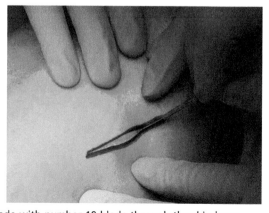

Fig. 8. Incision made with number 10 blade through the skin layer.

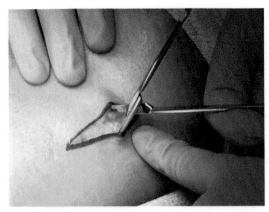

Fig. 9. Metzenbaum scissors used to dissect to the level of the deep fascia.

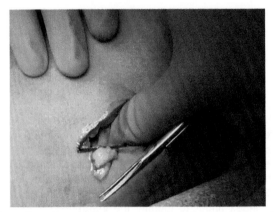

Fig. 10. Digital blunt dissection used to expose the deep fascia overlying the gastrocnemius and soleus muscles.

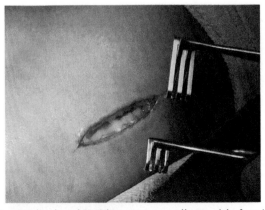

Fig. 11. Chung retractor (*top*) and Weitlaner retractor (*bottom*) before insertion for exposure of the deep fascial layer.

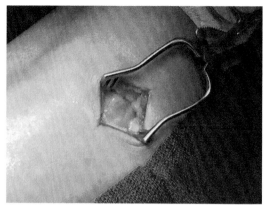

Fig. 12. Chung retractor in place to expose deep fascia overlying the gastrocnemius and soleus muscles.

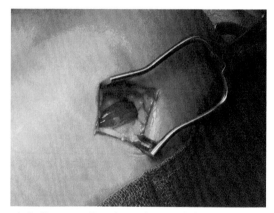

Fig. 13. Soleus muscle belly protruding through incised deep fascia.

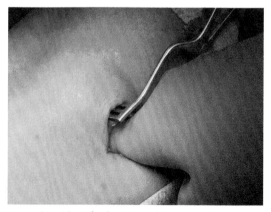

Fig. 14. Index finger used to identify the interval between the gastrocnemius and soleus muscles.

Step 7. An anal speculum is inserted between the gastrocnemius (posterior) and soleus (anterior) muscle bellies to expose the fascial layers of both muscles. The fascial layer is superior to the conjoined aponeurosis of the muscles (**Figs. 15** and **16**).

Step 8. A long-handled 15 blade is used to incise the gastrocnemius fascial layer from lateral to medial along the distal aspect of the anal speculum. Care must be taken to avoid cutting into the muscle of the gastrocnemius too deeply. It is important to incise the intermuscular septum between the medial and lateral heads of the gastrocnemius muscle. If present, the plantaris muscle is identified (usually along the soleus side) and released as well (**Fig. 17**).

Step 9. Ankle joint dorsiflexion is checked with the knee extended and the foot supinated. If ankle joint dorsiflexion is greater than 5° with the knee extended, then no further release is required. If ankle joint dorsiflexion is less than 5°, then a second recession is recommended of the gastrocnemius fascial layer approximately 1 cm proximal to the first recession (**Figs. 18** and **19**).

Step 10. Reapproximation of the deep fascia is with a 3-0 absorbable suture after irrigation of the surgical site. The author prefers to use 10 mL of 0.5% Marcaine with epinephrine as irrigation for this procedure. Closure of this layer is important to avoid the muscles herniating out of the medial calf during ambulation and producing a cosmetically poor result (**Fig. 20**).

Step 11. Skin closure is with 4-0 nylon sutures. The author uses an amniotic membrane product during skin closure to reduce the postoperative inflammatory response and thereby reduce postoperative wound dehiscence.

COMPLICATIONS AND MANAGEMENT

Equinus recurrence rates for GR are from 10% to 35% in the literature.[137,156,157] Specifically for the Baumann procedure, recurrence rates have been documented as approximately 10% for nonneurologic patients and 24% of neurologic patients.[137,157] Because of this high deformity recurrence rate, postprocedure bracing should be considered. The use of an equinus-type brace for 8 to 12 weeks once complete healing has occurred could help prevent recurrence.

Wound and subsequent scar complications, and weakness leading to overcorrection, seem to be minor compared with TALs and Strayer GR.[137,155,157,158]

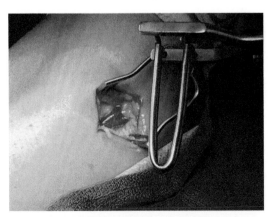

Fig. 15. Anal speculum before insertion between the gastrocnemius and soleus muscles. Note the soleus muscle protruding through the incised fascia.

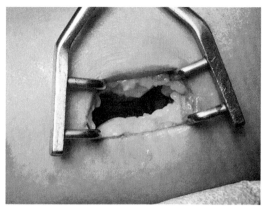

Fig. 16. Anal speculum in place distracting gastrocnemius and soleus fascial layers.

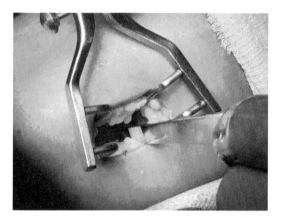

Fig. 17. Long-handle 15 blade used to cut the gastrocnemius fascial layer from lateral to medial at the distal aspect of the anal speculum.

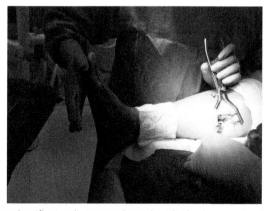

Fig. 18. Ankle joint dorsiflexion being evaluated with the knee extended after the initial recession of the gastrocnemius fascial layer.

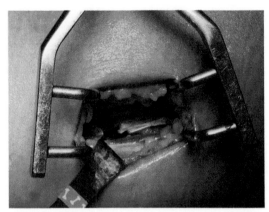

Fig. 19. Gastrocnemius fascial layer incised showing gapping between the proximal and distal ends.

POSTOPERATIVE CARE

Typically, a Baumann GR is done in combination with other procedures that establish the postoperative protocol. For patients undergoing only a Baumann GR, assisted weight-bearing in a cast brace for 2 weeks is a standard postoperative approach.[63] Transition to an athletic shoe with regular daily walking is allowed for the next 4 weeks. After 6 weeks, patients may return to their normal activity levels, and shoe gear is permitted.

OUTCOMES

Herzenberg and colleagues[153] examined the amount of correction obtained with various recessions of the gastrocnemius and soleus muscles and complete Achilles tenotomy (**Table 4**). The study showed that a second GR produced more ankle joint dorsiflexion than a soleus recession, which corresponds with Baumann and Koch's[151,152] original description of multiple gastrocnemius recessions.[151–153] Saraph and colleagues'[154] results for the Baumann GR in children with cerebral palsy showed significant

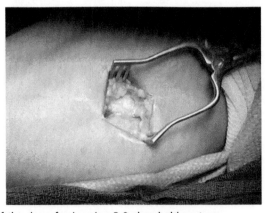

Fig. 20. Closure of the deep fascia using 3-0 absorbable suture.

Table 4					
Results of Herzenberg and colleagues'[153] study on Baumann gastrocnemius recession					
	Preoperative	First GR	Second GR	Soleus Recession	Achilles Tenotomy
AJ DF with Knee Extended	1°	9°	15°	16°	25°
AJ DF with Knee Flexed	12°	17°	20°	21°	27°

Abbreviation: AJ, ankle joint.
Data from Herzenberg J, Lamm B, Corwin C, et al. Isolated recession of the gastrocnemius muscle: the Baumann procedure. Foot Ankle Int 2007;28(11):1154–9.

improvement in active and passive ankle joint dorsiflexion with the knee extended and flexed, without any decrease in ankle joint plantarflexion power. Similarly, Rong and colleagues's[137] study on the Baumann GR for adult and pediatric flatfoot reconstruction resulted in 13.6° of increased ankle joint dorsiflexion with the knee extended and 9.7° with the knee flexed. Rong and colleagues[137] noted no weakness postoperatively. In addition, Svehlík and colleagues[155] evaluated the Baumann GR to correct equinus in children with diplegic cerebral palsy, showing significant improvement in ankle joint kinematics without weakness over the course of the 10-year follow-up.

SUMMARY

The literature is clear regarding equinus and its pathologic influence on the lower extremity. The multitude of associated lower extremity disorders linked to equinus in the literature provides solid evidence for including the treatment of equinus as part of any global treatment. Barouk[159] described the importance of equinus possibly more profoundly than any other author on the topic:

Looking for a retraction of the gastrocnemius should be an essential part of the foot and ankle examination for practitioners, not just surgeons. Even though the equinus has been recognized for 50 years as having an influence on the foot, only a few practitioners routinely search for it. The proportion of gastrocnemius tightness is high in the normal population, but it is significantly higher in populations that have foot and ankle problems.

I hope you will be convinced of the importance of this, and no longer do without!

REFERENCES

1. Hill R. Ankle equinus. Prevalence and linkage to common foot pathology. J Am Podiatr Med Assoc 1995;85(6):295–300.
2. DiGiovanni C, Kuo R, Tejwani N, et al. Isolated gastrocnemius tightness. J Bone Joint Surg Am 2002;84(6):962–70.
3. Lundgren P, Nester C, Liu A, et al. Invasive in vivo measurement of rear-, mid- and forefoot motion during walking. Gait Posture 2008;28(1):93–100.
4. Evans A, Scutter S. Sagittal plane range of motion of the pediatric ankle joint. J Am Podiatr Med Assoc 2006;96(5):418–22.
5. Pate AD, Giovanni B. Association between plantar fasciitis and isolated contracture of the gastrocnemius. Foot Ankle Int 2011;32(01):5–8.
6. Maskill J, Bohay D, Anderson J. Gastrocnemius recession to treat isolated foot pain. Foot Ankle Int 2010;31(01):19–23.

7. Singh D, Angel J, Bentley G, et al. Fortnightly review: plantar fasciitis. BMJ 1997; 315(7101):172–5.
8. Kibler W, Goldberg C, Chandler T. Functional biomechanical deficits in running athletes with plantar fasciitis. Am J Sports Med 1991;19(1):66–71.
9. Riddle D, Pulisic M, Pidcoe P, et al. Risk factors for plantar fasciitis: a matched case-control study. J Bone Joint Surg Am 2003;85(5):872–7.
10. Stotler W, Van Bergeyk A, Manoli A. Preliminary results of gastrocnemius recession in adults with nonspastic equinus contracture. In: American Orthopaedic Foot And Ankle Society 18th Annual Summer Meeting. Traverse City, MI, July 12–14, 2002.
11. Verrall G, Schofield S, Brustad T. Chronic Achilles tendinopathy treated with eccentric stretching program. Foot Ankle Int 2011;32(09):843–9.
12. Amis J. The gastrocnemius. Foot Ankle Clin 2014;19(4):637–47.
13. Gurdezi S, Kohls-Gatzoulis J, Solan M. Results of proximal medial gastrocnemius release for Achilles tendinopathy. Foot Ankle Int 2013;34(10):1364–9.
14. Alvarez R, Marini A, Schmitt C, et al. Stage I and II posterior tibial tendon dysfunction treated by a structured nonoperative management protocol: an orthosis and exercise program. Foot Ankle Int 2006;27(1):2–8.
15. Aronow M. Triceps surae contractures associated with posterior tibial tendon dysfunction. Tech Orthop 2000;15(3):164–73.
16. Downey MS, Banks AS. Gastrocnemius recession in the treatment of nonspastic ankle equinus. A retrospective study. J Am Podiatr Med Assoc 1989;79(4): 159–74.
17. Harris R, Beath T. Hypermobile flatfoot with short tendo Achilles. J Bone Joint Surg Am 1948;30(1):116–50.
18. Hibbs R. Muscle bound feet. NY Med J 1914;17(C):797–9.
19. Hoke M. An operation for the correction of extremely relaxed flat feet. J Bone Joint Surg 1931;13(4):773–83.
20. Sgarlato T, Morgan J, Shane H, et al. Tendo achillis lengthening and its effect on foot disorders. J Am Podiatr Med Assoc 1975;65(9):849–71.
21. Kaufman K, Brodine S, Shaffer R, et al. The effect of foot structure and range of motion on musculoskeletal overuse injuries. Am J Sports Med 1999;27(5): 585–93.
22. Wilder R, Sethi S. Overuse injuries: tendinopathies, stress fractures, compartment syndrome, and shin splints. Clin Sports Med 2004;23(1):55–81.
23. Ekstrand J, Gillquist J. The frequency of muscle tightness and injuries in soccer players. Am J Sports Med 1982;10(2):75–8.
24. Neely F. Biomechanical risk factors for exercise-related lower limb injuries. Sports Med 1998;26(6):395–413.
25. Messier SP, Pittala KA. Etiologic factors associated with selected running injuries. Med Sci Sports Exerc 1988;20(5):501–5.
26. Lun V. Relation between running injury and static lower limb alignment in recreational runners. Br J Sports Med 2004;38(5):576–80.
27. Tabrizi P, McIntyre W, Quesnel M, et al. Limited dorsiflexion predisposes to injuries of the ankle in children. J Bone Joint Surg 2000;82(8):1103–6.
28. Armstrong D, Stacpoole-Shea S, Nguyen H, et al. Lengthening of the Achilles tendon in diabetic patients who are at high risk for ulceration of the foot. J Bone Joint Surg 1999;81(4):535–8.
29. Barry D, Sabacinski K, Habershaw G, et al. Tendo Achillis procedures for chronic ulcerations in diabetic patients with transmetatarsal amputations. J Am Podiatr Med Assoc 1993;83(2):96–100.

30. Lin S, Lee T, Wapner K. Plantar forefoot ulceration with equinus deformity of the ankle in diabetic patients: the effect of tendo-Achilles lengthening and total contact casting. Orthopedics 1996;19(5):465–75.
31. Mueller M, Sinacore D, Hastings M, et al. Effect of Achilles tendon lengthening on neuropathic plantar ulcers. A randomized clinical trial. J Bone Joint Surg Am 2003;85(8):1436–45.
32. Nishimoto G, Attinger C, Cooper P. Lengthening the Achilles tendon for the treatment of diabetic plantar forefoot ulceration. Surg Clin North Am 2003;83(3): 707–26.
33. Early J, Hansen S. Surgical reconstruction of the diabetic foot: a salvage approach for midfoot collapse. Foot Ankle Int 1996;17(6):325–30.
34. Schon L, Easley M, Weinfeld B. Charcot neuroarthropathy of the foot and ankle. Clin Orthop Relat Res 1998;349:116–31.
35. Hansen S. Functional reconstruction of the foot and ankle. Philadelphia: Lippincott Williams & Wilkins; 2000.
36. Subotnick S. Equinus deformity as it affects the forefoot. J Am Podiatr Med Assoc 1971;61(11):423–7.
37. Banks A, McGlamry E. Charcot foot. J Am Podiatr Med Assoc 1989;79:213–35.
38. McGlamry E, Banks AS. McGlamry's comprehensive textbook of foot and ankle surgery. Philadelphia: Lippincott Williams & Wilkins; 2001.
39. Grant W, Sullivan R, Sonenshine D, et al. Electron microscopic investigation of the effects of diabetes mellitus on the Achilles tendon. J Foot Ankle Surg 1997;36(4):272–8.
40. Hansen S. Hallux valgus surgery. Morton and Lapidus were right. Clin Podiatr Med Surg 1996;13:347–54.
41. Barouk P, Barouk L. Clinical diagnosis of gastrocnemius tightness. Foot Ankle Clin 2014;19(9):659–67.
42. Jordan R, Cooper M, Schuster R. Ankle dorsiflexion at the heel-off phase of gait: a photokinegraphic study. J Am Podiatr Med Assoc 1979;69(1):40–6.
43. Lavery L, Armstrong D, Boulton A. Ankle equinus deformity and its relationship to high plantar pressure in a large population with diabetes mellitus. J Am Podiatr Med Assoc 2002;92(9):479–82.
44. Green D, Ruch J, McGlamry E. Correction of equinus-related forefoot deformities: a case report. J Am Podiatr Med Assoc 1976;66(10):768–80.
45. Root M, Orien W, Weed J. Normal and abnormal function of the foot. Los Angeles (CA): Clinical Biomechanics Corp.; 1977. p. 165–79, 295.
46. Lilletvedt J, Kreighbaum E, Phillips R. Analysis of selected alignment of the lower extremity related to the shin splint syndrome. J Am Podiatr Med Assoc 1979;69(3):211–7.
47. Pope R, Herbert R, Kirwan J. Effects of ankle dorsiflexion range and preexercise calf muscle stretching on injury risk in army recruits. Aust J Physiother 1998;44(3):165–72.
48. Fredericson M. Common injuries in runners. Sports Med 1996;21(1):49–72.
49. Gajdosik R, Vander Linden D, McNair P, et al. Effects of an eight-week stretching program on the passive-elastic properties and function of the calf muscles of older women. Clin Biomech 2005;20(9):973–83.
50. Becerro de Bengoa Vallejo R, Losa Iglesias M, Rodriguez Sanz D, et al. Plantar pressures in children with and without Sever's disease. J Am Podiatr Med Assoc 2011;101(1):17–24.
51. Szames S, Forman W, Oster J, et al. Sever's disease and its relationship to equinus: a statistical analysis. Clin Podiatr Med Surg 1990;7(2):377–84.

52. Holstein A. Hallux valgus–an acquired deformity of the foot in cerebral palsy. Foot Ankle Int 1980;1(1):33–8.
53. Nemec S, Habbu R, Anderson J, et al. Outcomes following midfoot arthrodesis for primary arthritis. Foot Ankle Int 2011;32(04):355–61.
54. Reimers J, Pedersen B, Brodersen A. Foot deformity and the length of the triceps surae in Danish children between 3 and 17 years old. J Pediatr Orthop B 1995;4(1):71–3.
55. DiGiovanni C, Langer P. The role of isolated gastrocnemius and combined Achilles contractures in the flatfoot. Foot Ankle Clin 2007;12(2):363–79.
56. Gourdine-Shaw M, Lamm B, Herzenberg J, et al. Equinus deformity in the pediatric patient: causes, evaluation, and management. Clin Podiatr Med Surg 2010; 27(1):25–42.
57. Lamm B, Paley D, Herzenberg J. Gastrocnemius soleus recession. J Am Podiatr Med Assoc 2005;95(1):18–25.
58. Powell M, Post W, Keener J, et al. Effective treatment of chronic plantar fasciitis with dorsiflexion night splints: a crossover prospective randomized outcome study. Foot Ankle Int 1998;19(1):10–8.
59. Wapner K, Sharkey P. The use of night splints for treatment of recalcitrant plantar fasciitis. Foot Ankle Int 1991;12(3):135–7.
60. Batt M, Tanji J, Skattum N. Plantar fasciitis: a prospective randomized clinical trial of the tension night splint. Clin J Sport Med 1996;6(3):158–62.
61. Lee W, Wong W, Kung E, et al. Effectiveness of adjustable dorsiflexion night splint in combination with accommodative foot orthosis on plantar fasciitis. J Rehabil Res Dev 2012;49(10):1557.
62. Abbassian A, Kohls-Gatzoulis J, Solan M. Proximal medial gastrocnemius release in the treatment of recalcitrant plantar fasciitis. Foot Ankle Int 2012; 33(1):14–9.
63. Monteagudo M, Maceira E, Garcia-Virto V, et al. Chronic plantar fasciitis: plantar fasciotomy versus gastrocnemius recession. Int Orthop 2013;37(9):1845–50.
64. Pascual Huerta J. The effect of the gastrocnemius on the plantar fascia. Foot Ankle Clin 2014;19(4):701–18.
65. Barouk L. The effect of gastrocnemius tightness on the pathogenesis of juvenile hallux valgus. Foot Ankle Clin 2014;19(4):807–22.
66. Beyzadeoglu T, Gokce A, Bekler H. The effectiveness of dorsiflexion night splint added to conservative treatment for plantar fasciitis. Acta Orthop Traumatol Turc 2007;41(3):220–4 [in Turkish].
67. Maceira E, Monteagudo M. Functional hallux rigidus and the Achilles-calcaneus-plantar system. Foot Ankle Clin 2014;19(4):669–99.
68. Solan M, Carne A, Davies M. Gastrocnemius shortening and heel pain. Foot Ankle Clin 2014;19(4):719–38.
69. Porter D, Barrill E, Oneacre K, et al. The effects of duration and frequency of Achilles tendon stretching on dorsiflexion and outcome in painful heel syndrome: a randomized, blinded, control study. Foot Ankle Int 2002;23(7):619–24.
70. Bolívar Y, Munuera P, Padillo J. Relationship between tightness of the posterior muscles of the lower limb and plantar fasciitis. Foot Ankle Int 2013;34(1):42–8.
71. Sheridan L, Lopez A, Perez A, et al. Plantar fasciopathy treated with dynamic splinting. J Am Podiatr Med Assoc 2010;100(3):161–5.
72. DiGiovanni B, Moore A, Zlotnicki J, et al. Preferred management of recalcitrant plantar fasciitis among orthopaedic foot and ankle surgeons. Foot Ankle Int 2012;33(6):507–12.

73. Davis P, Severud E, Baxter D. Painful heel syndrome: results of nonoperative treatment. Foot Ankle Int 1994;15(10):531–5.
74. Labovitz J, Yu J, Kim C. The role of hamstring tightness in plantar fasciitis. Foot Ankle Spec 2011;4(3):141–4.
75. Flanigan R, Nawoczenski D, Chen L, et al. The influence of foot position on stretching of the plantar fascia. Foot Ankle Int 2007;28(7):815–22.
76. Kiewiet N, Holthusen S, Bohay D, et al. Gastrocnemius recession for chronic noninsertional Achilles tendinopathy. Foot Ankle Int 2013;34(4):481–5.
77. Phisitkul P, Rungprai C, Femino J, et al. Endoscopic gastrocnemius recession for the treatment of isolated gastrocnemius contracture: a prospective study on 320 consecutive patients. Foot Ankle Int 2014;35(8):747–56.
78. Chen L, Greisberg J. Achilles lengthening procedures. Foot Ankle Clin 2009; 14(4):627–37.
79. Konrad A, Tilp M. Increased range of motion after static stretching is not due to changes in muscle and tendon structures. Clin Biomech 2014;29(6):636–42.
80. Ryan E, Beck T, Herda T, et al. The time course of musculotendinous stiffness responses following different durations of passive stretching. J Orthop Sports Phys Ther 2008;38(10):632–9.
81. Mahieu N, McNair P, De Muynck M, et al. Effect of static and ballistic stretching on the muscle-tendon tissue properties. Med Sci Sports Exerc 2007;39(3): 494–501.
82. Guissard N, Duchateau J. Effect of static stretch training on neural and mechanical properties of the human plantar-flexor muscles. Muscle Nerve 2004;29(2): 248–55.
83. Nakamura M, Ikezoe T, Takeno Y, et al. Effects of a 4-week static stretch training program on passive stiffness of human gastrocnemius muscle-tendon unit in vivo. Eur J Appl Physiol 2012;112(7):2749–55.
84. Macklin K, Healy A, Chockalingam N. The effect of calf muscle stretching exercises on ankle joint dorsiflexion and dynamic foot pressures, force and related temporal parameters. Foot 2012;22(1):10–7.
85. Aronow A, Diaz-Doran V, Sullivan R, et al. The effect of triceps surae contracture force on plantar foot pressure distribution. Foot Ankle Int 2006;27(1):43–52.
86. Goldsmith J, Lidtke R, Shott S. The effects of range-of-motion therapy on the plantar pressures of patients with diabetes mellitus. J Am Podiatr Med Assoc 2002;92(9):483–90.
87. Johanson M, DeArment A, Hines K, et al. The effect of subtalar joint position on dorsiflexion of the ankle/rearfoot versus midfoot/forefoot during gastrocnemius stretching. Foot Ankle Int 2013;35(1):63–70.
88. Mecagni C, Smith J, Roberts K, et al. Balance and ankle range of motion in community-dwelling women aged 64 to 87 years: a correlational study. Phys Ther 2000;80(10):1004–11.
89. Johnson E, Bradley B, Witkowski K, et al. Effect of a static calf muscle-tendon unit stretching program on ankle dorsiflexion range of motion of older women. J Geriatr Phys Ther 2007;30(2):49–52.
90. Rogers Mevans W. Changes in skeletal muscle with aging. Exerc Sport Sci Rev 1993;21(1):65–102.
91. Nurmi I, Lüthje P. Incidence and costs of falls and fall injuries among elderly in institutional care. Scand J Prim Health Care 2002;20(2):118–22.
92. Fuller G. Falls in the elderly. Am Fam Physician 2000;61(7):2159–68.

93. Gadjosik R, Vander Linden D, Williams A. Influence of age on length and passive elastic stiffness characteristics of the calf muscle-tendon unit of women. Phys Ther 1999;79:827–38.
94. Radford J, Burns J, Buchbinder R, et al. Does stretching increase ankle dorsiflexion range of motion? A systematic review. Br J Sports Med 2006;40(10): 870–5.
95. Bohannon R, Tiberio D, Zito M. Effect of five minute stretch on ankle dorsiflexion range of motion. J Phys Ther Sci 1994;6:1–8.
96. Knight C, Rutledge C, Cox M, et al. Effect of superficial heat, deep heat, and active exercise warm-up on the extensibility of the plantar flexors. Phys Ther 2001;81(6):1206–14.
97. Peres S, Draper D, Knight K, et al. Pulsed shortwave diathermy and prolonged long-duration stretching increase dorsiflexion range of motion more than identical stretching without diathermy. J Athl Train 2002;37(1):43.
98. Pratt K, Bohannon R. Effects of a 3-minute standing stretch on ankle-dorsiflexion range of motion. Trial 2003;2:80–5.
99. Evans A. Podiatric medical applications of posterior night stretch splinting. J Am Podiatr Med Assoc 2001;91:356–60.
100. Barry L, Barry A, Chen Y. A retrospective study of standing gastrocnemius-soleus stretching versus night splinting in the treatment of plantar fasciitis. J Foot Ankle Surg 2002;41(4):221–7.
101. Cheng H, Ju Y, Lin C. Design and validation of a dynamic stretch splint for plantar fasciitis. Med Eng Phys 2012;34(7):920–8.
102. Roos E, Engström M, Söderberg B. Foot orthoses for the treatment of plantar fasciitis. Foot Ankle Int 2006;27(8):606–11.
103. Kay A, Blazevich A. Moderate-duration static stretch reduces active and passive plantar flexor moment but not Achilles tendon stiffness or active muscle length. J Appl Physiol 2009;106(4):1249–56.
104. Grady J, Saxena A. Effects of stretching the gastrocnemius muscle. J Foot Surg 1990;30(5):465–9.
105. Chadchavalpanichaya N, Srisawasdi G, Suwannakin A. The effect of calf stretching box on stretching calf muscle compliance: a prospective, randomized single-blinded controlled trial. J Med Assoc Thai 2010;93(12):1470–9.
106. Youdas J, Krause D, Egan K, et al. The effect of static stretching of the calf muscle-tendon unit on active ankle dorsiflexion range of motion. J Orthop Sports Phys Ther 2003;33(7):408–17.
107. Zito M, Driver D, Parker C, et al. Lasting effects of one bout of two 15-second passive stretches on ankle dorsiflexion range of motion. J Orthop Sports Phys Ther 1997;26(4):214–21.
108. Young R, Nix S, Wholohan A, et al. Interventions for increasing ankle joint dorsiflexion: a systematic review and meta-analysis. J Foot Ankle Res 2013;6(1):46.
109. Berlet G, Anderson R, Davis W, et al. A prospective trial of night splinting in the treatment of recalcitrant plantar fasciitis: the Ankle Dorsiflexion Dynasplint. Orthopedics 2002;25(11):1273–5.
110. Manal K, Roberts D, Buchanan T. Optimal pennation angle of the primary ankle plantar and dorsiflexors: variations with sex, contraction intensity, and limb. J Appl Biomech 2006;22(4):255.
111. Abellaneda S, Guissard N, Duchateau J. The relative lengthening of the myotendinous structures in the medial gastrocnemius during passive stretching differs among individuals. J Appl Physiol 2008;106(1):169–77.

112. Levangie P, Norkin C. Joint structure and function: a comprehensive analysis. 2nd edition. Philadelphia: FA Davis; 2011.

113. Murray M, Kory R, Clarkson B, et al. Comparison of free and fast speed walking patterns of normal men. Am J Phys Med Rehabil 1966;45(1):8–24.

114. Karas M, Hoy D. Compensatory midfoot dorsiflexion in the individual with heel-cord tightness: implications for orthotic device designs. J Prosthetics Orthotics 2002;14(2):82–93.

115. Riemann B, DeMont R, Ryu K, et al. The effects of sex, joint angle, and the gastrocnemius muscle on passive ankle joint complex stiffness/commentary/author's response. J Athl Train 2001;36(4):369.

116. Johnson Christensen J. Biomechanics of the first ray part V: the effect of equinus deformity. J Foot Ankle Surg 2005;44(2):114–20.

117. Mueller M. The ankle and foot complex joint structure & function. Philadelphia: FA Davis; 2005. p. 437–77.

118. Caruntu D, Hefzy M. 3-D anatomically based dynamic modeling of the human knee to include tibio-femoral and patello-femoral joints. J Biomech Eng 2004; 126(1):44.

119. Moglo K, Shirazi-Adl A. Cruciate coupling and screw-home mechanism in passive knee joint during extension–flexion. J Biomech 2005;38(5):1075–83.

120. Frykberg R, Bowen J, Hall J, et al. Prevalence of equinus in diabetic versus nondiabetic patients. J Am Podiatr Med Assoc 2012;102(2):84–8.

121. Zimny S, Schatz H, Pfohl M. The role of limited joint mobility in diabetic patients with an at-risk foot. Diabetes Care 2004;27(4):942–6.

122. Greenhagen R, Johnson A, Bevilacqua N. Gastrocnemius recession or tendo-Achilles lengthening for equinus deformity in the diabetic foot? Clin Podiatr Med Surg 2012;29(3):413–24.

123. Barrett S, Jarvis J. Equinus deformity as a factor in forefoot nerve entrapment. J Am Podiatr Med Assoc 2005;95(5):464–8.

124. Chimera N, Castro M, Manal K. Function and strength following gastrocnemius recession for isolated gastrocnemius contracture. Foot Ankle Int 2010;31(5): 377–84.

125. Chimera N, Castro M, Davis I, et al. The effect of isolated gastrocnemius contracture and gastrocnemius recession on lower extremity kinematics and kinetics during stance. Clin Biomech 2012;27(9):917–23.

126. Pinney S, Hansen S, Sangeorzan B. The effect on ankle dorsiflexion of gastrocnemius recession. Foot Ankle Int 2002;23(1):26–9.

127. Duthon V, Lübbeke A, Duc S, et al. Noninsertional Achilles tendinopathy treated with gastrocnemius lengthening. Foot Ankle Int 2011;32(04):375–9.

128. Gentchos C, Bohay D, Anderson J. Gastrocnemius recession as treatment for refractory Achilles tendinopathy: a case report. Foot Ankle Int 2008;29(6):620–3.

129. Laborde J, Weiler L. Achilles tendon pain treated with gastrocnemius-soleus recession. Orthopedics 2011;34(4):289–91.

130. Dayer Rassal M. Chronic diabetic ulcers under the first metatarsal head treated by staged tendon balancing: a prospective cohort study. J Bone Joint Surg Br 2009;91(4):487–93.

131. Hamilton G, Ford L, Perez H, et al. Salvage of the neuropathic foot by using bone resection and tendon balancing: a retrospective review of 10 patients. J Foot Ankle Surg 2005;44(1):37–43.

132. Laborde J. Neuropathic plantar forefoot ulcers treated with tendon lengthenings. Foot Ankle Int 2008;29(4):378–84.

133. Laborde J. Midfoot ulcers treated with gastrocnemius-soleus recession. Foot Ankle Int 2009;30(9):842–6.

134. Cychosz C, Phisitkul P, Belatti D, et al. Gastrocnemius recession for foot and ankle conditions in adults: evidence-based recommendations. Foot Ankle Surg 2015;21(2):77–85.

135. Morales-Munoz P, De Los Santos Real R, Barrio Sanz P, et al. Gastrocnemius proximal release in the treatment of mechanical metatarsalgia: a prospective study of 78 cases. Foot Ankle Int 2016;37(7):782–9.

136. Nawoczenski D, DiLiberto F, Cantor M, et al. Ankle power and endurance outcomes following isolated gastrocnemius recession for Achilles tendinopathy. Foot Ankle Int 2016;37:766–75.

137. Rong K, Ge W, Li X, et al. Mid-term results of intramuscular lengthening of gastrocnemius and/or soleus to correct equinus deformity in flatfoot. Foot Ankle Int 2015;36(10):1223–8.

138. Nawoczenski D, Barske H, Tome J, et al. Isolated gastrocnemius recession for Achilles tendinopathy: strength and functional outcomes. J Bone Joint Surg 2015;97(2):99–105.

139. Tallerico V, Greenhagen R, Lowery C. Isolated gastrocnemius recession for treatment of insertional Achilles tendinopathy: a pilot study. Foot Ankle Spec 2014;8(4):260–5.

140. Phisitkul P. Endoscopic surgery of the Achilles tendon. Curr Rev Musculoskelet Med 2012;5(2):156–63.

141. Sammarco G, Bagwe M, Sammarco V, et al. The effects of unilateral gastrocsoleus recession. Foot Ankle Int 2006;27(7):508–11.

142. Elveru R, Rothstein J, Lamb R. Goniometric reliability in a clinical setting subtalar and ankle joint measurements. Phys Ther 1988;68(5):672–7.

143. Van Gheluwe B, Kirby K, Roosen P, et al. Reliability and accuracy of biomechanical measurements of the lower extremities. J Am Podiatr Med Assoc 2002; 92(6):317–26.

144. Martin R, McPoil T. Reliability of ankle goniometric measurements. J Am Podiatr Med Assoc 2005;95(6):564–72.

145. Thordarson D, Schmotzer H, Chon J, et al. Dynamic support of the human longitudinal arch. Clin Orthop Relat Res 1995;(316):165–72.

146. Nutt J. Diseases and deformities of the foot. New York: EB Treat & Company; 1913.

147. Salamon M, Pinney S, Van Bergeyk A, et al. Surgical anatomy and accuracy of percutaneous Achilles tendon lengthening. Foot Ankle Int 2006;27(6):411–3.

148. Holstein P, Lohmann M, Bitsch M, et al. Achilles tendon lengthening, the panacea for plantar forefoot ulceration? Diabetes Metab Res Rev 2004; 20(S1):S37–40.

149. Chilvers M, Malicky E, Anderson J, et al. Heel overload associated with heel cord insufficiency. Foot Ankle Int 2007;28(6):687–9.

150. Molund M, Paulsrud Ø, Ellingsen Husebye E, et al. Results after gastrocnemius recession in 73 patients. Foot Ankle Surg 2014;20(4):272–5.

151. Baumann J, Koch H. Ventrale aponeurotische Verlängerung des Musculus gastrocnemius. Oper Orthop Traumatol 1989;1(4):254–8.

152. Baumann J, Koch H. Lengthening of the anterior aponeurosis of musculus gastrocnemius through multiple incisions. Orthop Traumatol 1992;1(4):278–82.

153. Herzenberg J, Lamm B, Corwin C, et al. Isolated recession of the gastrocnemius muscle: the Baumann procedure. Foot Ankle Int 2007;28(11):1154–9.

154. Saraph V, Zwick E, Uitz C, et al. The Baumann procedure for fixed contracture of the gastrosoleus in cerebral palsy. J Bone Joint Surg 2000;82(4):535–40.
155. Svehlík M, Kraus T, Steinwender G, et al. The Baumann procedure to correct equinus gait in children with diplegic cerebral palsy: long-term results. Bone Joint J 2012;94B(8):1143–7.
156. Firth G, Passmore E, Sangeux M, et al. Multilevel surgery for equinus gait in children with spastic diplegic cerebral palsy. J Bone Joint Surg Am 2013; 95(10):931.
157. Dreher T, Buccoliero T, Wolf S, et al. Long-term results after gastrocnemius-soleus intramuscular aponeurotic recession as a part of multilevel surgery in spastic diplegic cerebral palsy. J Bone Joint Surg Am 2012;94(7):627–37.
158. El-Adwar K, Abdul-Rahman E, Al-Magrabri E. The treatment of fixed contracture of the gastrosoleus in cerebral palsy using the Baumann procedure: preliminary results of a prospective study. Curr Orthop Pract 2009;20(4):448–53.
159. Barouk P. Introduction to gastrocnemius tightness. Foot Ankle Clin 2014; 19(4):xv.

Acute Achilles Tendon Rupture

Clinical Evaluation, Conservative Management, and Early Active Rehabilitation

Merrell Kauwe, DPM

KEYWORDS

- Functional rehabilitation • Nonsurgical treatment • Postsurgical rehabilitation

KEY POINTS

- History and physical examination is the cornerstone for acute Achilles tendon rupture. Imaging is rarely needed for diagnosis, as physical examination is highly sensitive and specific.
- Conservative treatment provides the same outcome as surgical treatment without the risk of surgery, but only when functional rehabilitation protocols are used.
- There remains variability in reported functional rehabilitation protocols, although it is clear that early weight bearing with controlled early range of motion improve patient satisfaction and outcome.
- Regardless of conservative or surgical treatment, functional rehabilitation should be used.

INTRODUCTION

The Achilles tendon (AT) is the strongest and largest tendon in the human body. It is also the most frequently ruptured. The incidence of rupture has reportedly risen over time.[1–4] Increase in incidence is often attributed to increasing elderly and obese populations as well as increase in recreation sporting activities by middle-aged individuals.[5] Investigations into etiology have observed multiple factors that may be contributory to primary AT rupture.

Treatment of AT rupture remains controversial as risk and benefits of conservative versus surgical repair continue to be debated.[6] The conclusions of most early studies observing surgical versus conservative treatment were that surgery provides lower risk of re-rupture with higher complication rates.[7–13] Conservative treatment has gained increasing support with the advent of functional rehabilitation protocols, with

Foot and Ankle Department, UnityPoint Trinity Regional Medical Center, 804 Kenyon Road, Suite 310, Fort Dodge, IA 50501, USA
E-mail address: merrellkauwe@gmail.com

Clin Podiatr Med Surg 34 (2017) 229–243
http://dx.doi.org/10.1016/j.cpm.2016.10.009
0891-8422/17/© 2016 Elsevier Inc. All rights reserved.
podiatric.theclinics.com

more recent studies concluding that nonoperative treatment with functional rehabilitation is preferred. It leads to similar re-rupture rates and functional outcomes as surgery, with decreased complications.[14–18] Functional rehabilitation in the postoperative setting has also increased over the past few decades with studies suggesting it can reduce time to return to normal activities, increase patient satisfaction, and improve functional outcome.

EPIDEMIOLOGY AND ETIOLOGY OF RUPTURE

Incidence rates of AT rupture range from 11 to 37 per 100,00 population.[19–23] Gender distribution is predominately male with a reported male-female ratio ranging from 2:1 to 12:1.[24] Epidemiologic studies show an increase peak in incidence in middle-aged (30–39 years) individuals with AT rupture related to sports injuries and a second smaller peak due to other causes in later in life. Moller and colleagues[25] and Nillius and colleagues[26] showed the second peak to occur in the eighth decade of life, whereas Leppilahti and colleagues[21] reported the second peak distribution in the fifth decade.

Rupture of the AT most commonly occurs 3 to 6 cm proximal to the calcaneal insertion, with most injuries occurring during athletic activity.[27] The mechanism of injury is classified into 3 categories. First, weight bearing with the forefoot pushing off and the knee extended; second, an unanticipated dorsiflexion of the ankle; and third, a violent dorsiflexion of a plantarflexed foot.[28] Although the mechanism of rupture is observable, it is still unclear why the tendon itself ruptures and several theories have been advocated for. The location of rupture is partially explained by very high peak stresses experienced in this midportion area.[29] These stresses can lead to damage in tendons that are otherwise free of degenerative changes.[30]

It has been suggested that the failure of inhibitory mechanisms that would normally protect against excessive and/or uncoordinated muscle contractions could cause rupture at the site of maximum stress, and that athletes returning following inactivity may be particularly susceptible to this.[31]

Degenerative changes have been observed in AT ruptures. These changes can result from multiple factors, including chronic overloading and microtrauma, pharmacologic treatments, and reduced vascularity with associated heat necrosis.[32–39] Ischemia of the AT at the watershed zone has long been described as a factor in tendon rupture. This is despite recent experimental evidence showing uniform hemodynamic flow throughout the tendon at rest and at work. This is discussed in detail in this issue (See Paul Dayton's article, "Anatomic, Vascular, and Mechanical Overview of the Achilles Tendon," in this issue). It has been observed that corticosteroid use can cause degenerative tendon changes due to necrosis and delay in healing[40] and that the anti-inflammatory effect of steroids may mask painful symptoms of a damaged tendon, increasing the risk of rupture.[41] A study in 2004 by Gill and colleagues,[42] however, failed to show any causality between steroid injection for Achilles tendinopathy and AT rupture. Fluoroquinolones have been associated with AT degeneration and rupture as well. Multiple studies, including a cohort study of more than 6 million people, show increased risk for AT rupture with use.[43–47] Degenerative changes from fluoroquinolones likely follow from the drug's side effect of decreased decorin transcription.[33] Decorin is a small proteoglycan molecule that plays an important part in maintaining the molecular integrity of a tendon. Its decreased transcription is hypothesized to alter the viscoelastic properties of tendons and increase fragility.[39]

Claessen and colleagues,[48] in 2014, performed a systematic review to assess the many reported factors contributing to Achilles rupture. They identified nonmodifiable characteristics, such as age, race, gender, nonmusculoskeletal disease, trauma, pre-existing musculoskeletal disease, biomechanical foot and ankle position, and other genetic factors. They also identified modifiable factors, including obesity, hypercholesterolemia, sporting activities, medications including quinolones and corticosteroids, and other environmental factors. They found moderate evidence that decreased tendon fibril size increases AT rupture risk. Because tendon fibril size decreases with age, it is a risk factor as well.[49] All other factors had limited evidence, including body weight, corticosteroid use, and quinolone use.

Ischemia of the AT at the watershed zone has long been described as a factor in tendon rupture. This is despite recent experimental evidence showing uniform hemodynamic flow throughout the tendon at rest and at work. This is discussed in detail in this issue (See Paul Dayton's article, "Anatomic, Vascular, and Mechanical Overview of the Achilles Tendon," in this issue). Clearly there is a need for higher quality studies to establish determinants of AT rupture risk.

PATIENT EVALUATION OVERVIEW
History and Physical Evaluation

The patient history is generally straightforward, posing little diagnostic difficulty.[24] This is especially true in the cases of athletic activity in which patients report a pop, snap, or crack. They believe they have been hit or kicked or even shot in the area of the rupture. Although pain is immediate, it usually resolves quickly.[50] There is reported weakness, poor balance, and altered gait.[24] When the injury is not related to sporting activity or the injury is remote with poor history, AT rupture may be missed by physician and patient alike.[51] Inaccurate diagnosis can lead to chronic pain, swelling, poor gait, and inability to return to previous activity levels. This is concerning, as upward of 25% of the AT ruptures are missed,[51,52] usually diagnosed as ankle sprains.[53] Differential diagnosis for AT rupture includes AT peri-tendinitis, gastrocnemius tear, muscle strain or rupture, ligamentous injury, peroneal injury, and fracture.[50]

The physical examination of AT rupture can pose diagnostic problems. The patient may not report pain with examination of the tendon.[54] Although the AT is the major plantar flexor of the foot, plantarflexion weakness due to rupture can be masked by action of the posterior tibial, peroneal, and plantar muscles. In neglected ruptures, the extrinsic and intrinsic muscles of the foot may have assumed the role of foot plantarflexion, allowing the patient to walk into the examination room without exhibiting alteration of gait. This is also why the patient may exhibit passive and resisted plantarflexory strength during examination. Surrounding swelling and herniation of fat into the gap may make palpation of deficit difficult in an acute rupture. In neglected ruptures older than 4 weeks, the process of hematoma replacement with healing tendon tissue can "obliterate" the gap.[55]

Several diagnostic tests have been described to diagnose AT rupture. Understanding and use of these tests will help to minimize missed diagnoses. The calf-squeeze test, described by both Simmonds[56] in 1957 and Thompson[57] in 1962, is performed with the patient prone on the examination table with ankles clear of end of the table or with the knees flexed and feet hanging free at the end of a chair (**Fig. 1**).[36–58] The examiner squeezes the calf; doing so causes deformation of the soleus muscle with concurrent posterior bowstringing of the AT away from the tibia.[59] If there is plantarflexion of the foot, the test is negative and the tendon is intact. If the foot remains in neutral or there is minimal plantarflexion with comparison to the unaffected foot, the test is positive and there is a rupture of the AT. Maffulli[55] reported a sensitivity of 0.96 and specificity of 0.93 for the calf-squeeze test. False-negative for this test is

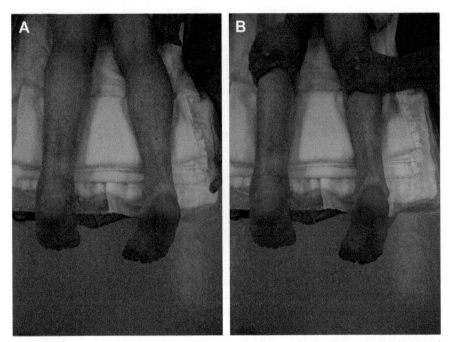

Fig. 1. This figure depicts the calf-squeeze test, also known as the Thompson or Simmonds test. It is performed while the patient is prone with the feet hanging off the edge of the table. The calf is squeezed causing a deforming bowstringing effect to the soleus, thereby plantarflexing the foot. (*A*) A resting state with acute AT rupture to the left lower extremity. (*B*) Execution of the calf-squeeze test. Note that there is little discernable plantarflexion of the foot of the affected left lower extremity while the contralateral limb exhibits an intact AT.

more likely with a neglected rupture in which hematoma has been replaced with healing tendon tissues.

The knee flexion test, also called the passive ankle dorsiflexion test, described my Matles in 1975,[60] is performed with the patient prone. The patient actively flexes the knee to 90°. The examiner observes both feet and ankles throughout flexion and with the tibia vertical. With an intact tendon, the examiner should observe slight plantarflexion. The affected foot will fall into neutral or dorsiflexion (**Fig. 2**). Maffulli[55] reported a sensitivity of 0.88 and specificity of 0.85 with this test. A neglected rupture should still be positive with the knee flexion test, as the tendon will lengthen with hematoma formation and subsequent tendon reconstitution.[55]

The sphygmomanometer test described by Copeland[61] is performed with the patient prone and a cuff placed around the middle calf. The cuff is inflated to 100 mm Hg with the ankle placed in position of passive plantar flexion by the examiner. With the examiner dorsiflexing the ankle an increase in pressure between 35 and 60 mm Hg is observed if the tendon is intact. If the tendon is ruptured, little or no pressure rise is seen. The needle test described by O'Brien[62] is performed with the patient under general or spinal anesthesia due to significant discomfort otherwise. A needle (21 gauge) is inserted at a right angle so that just the tip is within the substance of the tendon. It inserted through the skin medial to midline of calf and approximately 10 cm proximal to the superior portion of the calcaneus. The foot is then passively

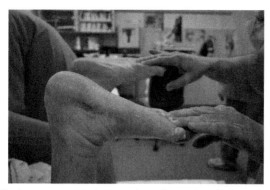

Fig. 2. The knee flexion test, or Matles test, is performed with the patient prone and the tibia brought to vertical. The affected lower extremity should show a neutral position or passive dorsiflexion when compared with the contralateral limb. In this image, we have added some dorsiflexory pressure to both extremities. Note the excessive amount of dorsiflexion present to the left lower extremity where there is an acute AT rupture with comparison to the right lower where the tendon is intact.

taken through dorsiflexion and plantarflexion range of motion. If the tendon is intact, the needle will swivel in opposite direction of the joint's position. If the needle does not move, or moves only slightly and in the direction, then the tendon has lost continuity with the insertion and rupture is likely. These 2 tests, the Copeland and O'Brien, had reported sensitivity by Maffulli[55] of 0.81 and 0.80 respectively with no specificities noted.

Reiman and colleagues[63] in 2014 performed a systematic review with meta-analysis of the utility of clinical measures for the diagnosis of tendon injuries. The calf-squeeze test had a positive likelihood ratio of 13.51 and a negative likelihood ratio of 0.04, giving in the ability to rule in or rule out an AT tear to a "large and almost conclusive degree." Maffulli[55] reports that the diagnosis of subcutaneous AT tear can reliably be diagnosed with a combination of the calf-squeeze and knee flexion test. The American Academy of Orthopaedic Surgeons (AAOS) requires findings consistent with rupture in 2 or more of the following tests for clinical diagnosis of AT rupture: calf-squeeze test, palpable gap, knee flexion test, or decreased plantarflexion strength.[64] Garras and colleagues[65] in a 2012 study comparing clinical examination with MRI for AT rupture showed a 100% sensitivity when the calf-squeeze, knee flexion test, and palpable defect were indicative of rupture. With such excellent sensitivity and specificity of easily performed diagnostic examinations, clinical examination is the standard for diagnosis.

Imaging Evaluation

Radiographs can be performed with the lateral ankle projections used to assess AT rupture. Attention should be paid to the Kager triangle. Loss of normal fat contours or soft tissue density within the normal radiopaque triangle may be suggestive of Achilles rupture. A positive Arner sign and a decreased Toygar angle are indicative of an AT rupture. A positive Arner sign is when the AT deviates anteriorly and no longer parallels the skin surface.[28] The Toygar angle is the ankle of the posterior skin adjacent to the AT. The angle of the skin at the posterior leg overlying the AT should be greater than 150°.[66]

Ultrasound has been described for use in assessment of AT rupture.[67–69] The recommended technique is performed with the patient in a prone position with the foot hanging off the edge of the table. The transducer should be at least 10 MHz, given the superficial location of the observed structures. The transducer should be placed in the sagittal plane with observation from the insertion into the calcaneus proximal to the myotendinous junction, then turned 90° for evaluation in the transverse plane. The AT should be uniform in thickness and echogenicity in the longitudinal plane. There should be a hypoechoic ribbonlike image between 2 hyperechoic bands. It should be predominately flat or have a concave anterior margin in the transverse plane. It is important to perform dynamic imaging when evaluating a rupture because fluid, debris, scar tissue, or hemorrhage may fill the gap between torn ends. This can be done by gently plantarflexing the foot or with the calf-squeeze test.[70] One typically observes an "acoustic vacuum" with thick irregular edges at the area of rupture.[71,72] When nonsurgical treatment is used, ultrasound imaging is a simple way to observe that the tendon ends are approximated when cast immobilization or functional bracing is positioned.

MRI is a useful imaging modality to study soft tissue injuries. Typically, the AT produces a hypointense signal with all imaging sequences. Almost all tears, complete and incomplete, show a high T2-weighted signal within the tendon and a focal area of signal intensity at the site of rupture where edema and hemorrhage have collected. Retraction of free ends can occur in acute AT tears with T1-weighted signal disruption throughout the tendon itself.[73] Garras and colleagues[65] performed a study to examine the sensitivity of physical examination and compare this to the sensitivity of MRI for assessment of AT rupture. In patients with calf-squeeze test, knee flexion test, and palpable gap test indicative of AT rupture, the findings were confirmed intraoperatively with a sensitivity of 100%. MRI study showed a sensitivity of 90%. Garras and colleagues[65] found that physical examination was more sensitive than MRI in diagnosing acute AT rupture. The AAOS describes use of imaging modalities, including radiograph, ultrasound, and MRI, to diagnose AT rupture as "inconclusive," meaning there is a lack of compelling evidence to support their use.[64] With such sensitive clinical examinations, it is recommended additional imaging be performed only when diagnosis with clinical findings is equivocal. This should be rarely, as diagnosis of acute AT rupture is based on clinical findings.

Conservative Versus Surgical Treatment

Management of AT rupture is dependent on surgeon and patient preference, with the aim of treatment to restore a normal-length tension relationship, optimizing strength and function while balancing these goals with the known complications of treatment.[6] Management options can be placed in the general categories of conservative and surgical treatment.

Multiple randomized controlled trials (RCTs) have been published comparing conservative and surgical treatment.[7,10,14,15,17,74–81] Multiple meta-analyses assessing these RCTs also have been published. Early RCTs before 2005,[7,10,74,78–80] as well as early meta-analyses assessing information before 2005,[82,83] show an increased risk of re-rupture with conservative treatment. Surgical treatment showed an increase in other complications, particularly skin healing and infection. After risk assessments, these meta-analyses recommended surgical treatment as the preferred method of addressing acute rupture. Subsequent RCTs, particularly those using functional bracing and dynamic or early active rehabilitation, produced results discordant with previous conclusions. They have found no difference in re-rupture rate.[14,17,74–77,81] Multiple meta-analyses have been published to assess these new and conflicting conclusions.[16,82–86]

In 2012, Soroceanu and colleagues[16] performed a meta-analysis including 10 RCTs. They found when functional rehabilitation with early range of motion were used, re-rupture rates for surgical and nonsurgical patients were equal without significant statistical difference (absolute risk difference 1.7%; $P = .45$). If such rehabilitation protocols were not used, surgery was favored due to increased re-rupture rates in the nonsurgical patients. They found there was no difference in calf circumference, strength, or functional outcomes between the groups when functional rehabilitation protocols were used, although surgery did provide a quicker return to work as well as a quicker return to previous activity levels. These functional protocols, including immediate weight bearing and mobilization as early as 10 days, stand in stark contrast to traditional conservative treatments of immobilization and non–weight bearing for 6 to 8 weeks. The traditional idea was thought to protect the surgical repair or maintain apposition of the tendon if conservative treatment was chosen. We know now that tendon repair is stimulated by mechanical loading.[87–91] Production of growth factors within the healing tendon are influenced by loading.[92] As little as 5 minutes of loading each day can improve the strength of healing tissues. This effect may be responsible for the decreased re-rupture rate when functional rehabilitation protocols are used in conservative care.

In 2015 Zhang and colleagues[93] published a systematic review of overlapping meta-analyses comparing conservative with surgical treatment. Nine meta-analyses were included. Their study found that when functional rehabilitation was used, conservative intervention was equal to surgical treatment regarding incidence of re-rupture, range of motion, calf circumference, and functional outcomes. They found incidence of other complications was reduced with conservative treatment. Their findings were agreement with Soroceanu and colleagues,[16] that when functional rehabilitation is not performed, conservative treatment significantly increased the re-rupture rate. From their study, they conclude that the best available evidence supports conservative intervention for AT rupture as the preferred treatment if there is access to functional rehabilitation. When this is not available, surgical treatment should be considered.

Regarding acceptable time frame on institution of conservative treatment protocols, there is no recommendation from the previously listed studies. Studies have varied from 3 to 14 days from injury to start of conservative treatment. It has been hypothesized that delay in conservative treatment of more than 14 days may prevent approximation of tendon ends, as scar tissues have developed at the gapped ends and the tendon is effectively lengthened.[94] It may be advisable to observe tendon ends under ultrasound to make sure they can approximate before initiating conservative treatment protocols.

EARLY ACTIVE REHABILITATION IN THE CONSERVATIVELY TREATED AND POSTSURGICAL PATIENT
Conservative Rehabilitation

Although early active rehabilitation has shown to benefit nonsurgical care, as evidenced by decreased re-rupture rate and good functional outcomes when used, the optimum protocol remains unclear. The various studies reporting on functional rehabilitation protocols for conservative treatment and following surgical intervention exhibit great heterogeneity. They vary in length of time immobilized, time to weight bearing, and orthosis type for functional care. These studies are primarily concerned about nonoperative and operative treatment comparisons, not on comparison of rehabilitation programs. Some prospective studies exist, but without control and multiple treatment groups, conclusions on which protocol is preferred are difficult.

In 2015, Hutchison and colleagues[95] reported on a series of 273 patients with acute AT rupture; 211 of these were managed conservatively, with 62 receiving surgical treatment. Re-rupture rate was reported at 1.1% for all. Conservative treatment and postsurgical treatment protocols were identical and included immediate weight bearing in fixed equinus position with immobilization until week 10. They used a specialized orthosis that had an adjustable ankle feature to set plantarflexion position as well as limit ankle dorsiflexion for controlled range of motion. All weight bearing was performed in the boot with progressive dorsiflexion to neutral. Ecker and colleagues,[96] in 2016, reported on 171 consecutive conservatively treated patients. Re-rupture rate was reported at 6.4%. Patients were casted in an equinus position, were fully weight bearing immediately, and remained immobilized for 6 weeks. They used a short-ankle rehabilitation boot with removable wedges for all weight bearing and progressively brought the foot from plantarflexed to neutral. Both of these studies used controlled early weight bearing in a fixed equinus with initial immobilization.

The study by Twaddle and Poon in 2007[17] used early mobilization with active ankle dorsiflexion and passive plantarflexion at 10 days in both surgical and nonsurgical groups alike. Although early weight bearing was not used, their study showed similar re-rupture rates and functional outcomes in the nonsurgical groups as did the studies by Ecker and colleagues[96] and Hutchison and colleagues[95] described previously in which prolonged immobilization occurred. Barfod and colleagues,[97] in 2014, published an RCT looking at the effect of weight bearing in conservative AT rupture care. They found immediate weight bearing with controlled early mobilization produced good functional outcomes and increased quality of life from when compared with non–weight bearing. Although early weight bearing alone appears to give good functional outcomes while limiting complications, a combination of both early weight bearing and controlled early mobilization may be best. **Table 1** provides a conservative treatment protocol.

Table 1
Rehabilitation protocol for conservative treatment of Achilles rupture

Time from Presentation, wk	Weight Bearing	Immobilization and Activity
0–2	Full weight bearing in orthosis in plantarflexion.	Immobilized in cast, splint, or boot with tendon ends opposed. This is generally 20°–30° of plantarflexion.
3–4	Full weight bearing with progressive reduction in plantarflexion.	Controlled early motion with legs freely hanging while performing active dorsiflexion to neutral and passive plantarflexion 5 minutes of every hour.
5–6	Full weight bearing with continued reduction in plantarflexion.	Continue controlled early motion as described above.
7–8	Full weight bearing in neutral position, no heel lift or plantarflexion.	Continue controlled early motion. Orthosis may be removed nightly.
9–12	Progressive individualized physical therapy working on strength, range of motion, proprioception. Review length of recovery expectations, including return to previous activity levels and sports.	

Adapted from Refs.[95–97]

Postsurgical Rehabilitation

Early functional rehabilitation has been the trend in postsurgical care as well is in conservative care. Delineating the roles of early mobilization and early weight bearing in postsurgical care carries with it similar difficulties in assessing conservative care protocols; specifically, there is heterogeneity within the literature.

To address this, Huang and colleagues[98] included 9 studies assessing postoperative rehabilitation in their published meta-analysis. Six of these studies included weight bearing with early ankle joint motion, whereas 3 used only early ankle joint motion without early weight bearing. They identified 15 functional outcome measures. Eleven of the 15 measures were better in the combined group when compared with traditional immobilization. Only 2 of the 14 measures were observed to be significantly better in the groups that performed only ankle joint range of motion when compared with traditional immobilization. They concluded that postoperative care should include combined early weight bearing with early ankle joint range of motion exercises.

In 2014, Brumann and colleagues[99] performed a systematic review to develop an evidence-based postoperative treatment protocol. They assessed full weight bearing versus non–weight bearing, early ankle mobilization versus immobilization, and combined functional treatment versus immobilization and non–weight bearing. Immediate full weight bearing led to earlier ambulation and return to previous activity levels as well as a significant increase in patient satisfaction versus non–weight bearing. Mobilization was shown to shorten time to return to work and sports to a significant level compared with immobilization. The combined early weight bearing and early ankle mobilization produced the best rehabilitation results with higher satisfaction, earlier return to work and preinjury activities, increased calf muscle strength, reduction in calf muscle atrophy and tendon elongation, and less use of resources. Not a single reviewed study showed an increase in rupture rate with early active rehabilitation protocols. Based on their review, Brumann and colleagues[99] recommend full weight bearing immediately after repair with the ankle fixed in 30° of plantar flexion with an orthosis. Range of motion should begin at week 3 with dorsiflexion to 0° and full plantarflexion allowed. Progressive reduction of weight-bearing plantarflexion should take place from weeks 3 to 6. At week 7, range of motion should be unrestricted with cessation of orthosis use. **Table 2** provides a postoperative functional rehabilitation protocol.

Table 2
Rehabilitation protocol for postsurgical treatment of Achilles rupture

Time from Surgery (wk)	Weight Bearing	Immobilization and Activity
0–2	Full weight bearing in orthosis in plantarflexion.	Immobilized in cast, splint, or orthosis at 30° plantarflexion.
3–6	Full weight bearing with progressive weekly reduction in plantarflexion of 10° per week until foot is at 0°.	Active mobilization of ankle from 0° dorsiflexion, with free range of motion in plantarflexion.
7+	Full weight bearing with no orthosis. Free range of motion. Individualized physical therapy to increase strength, range of motion, and proprioception.	

Adapted from Brumann M, Baumbach SF, Mutschler W, et al. Accelerated rehabilitation following Achilles tendon repair after acute rupture–development of an evidence based treatment protocol. Injury 2014;45:1782–90.

Regardless of operative or nonoperative treatment, a combination of immediate weight bearing with early ankle mobilization appears to be important for optimum patient recovery. Although there has been some attempt to understand the best course of rehabilitation, research remains to be performed to more clearly guide treatment measures in both settings.

SUMMARY

The incidence of AT rupture has trended up over the past few decades. Suspicion of AT rupture should remain high, as this diagnosis is frequently missed. Physical examination remains the cornerstone for diagnosis with high sensitivity and specificity. Additional imaging is not recommended unless examination findings are equivocal. Both conservative and surgical treatment provide good functional outcome when functional rehabilitation protocols are observed. Functional rehabilitation has lowered the risk of re-rupture with conservative care to the extent that there is no longer a significant difference in re-rupture rate compared with surgical treatment. Because of this lowered risk and the relative high complication risk of surgery, conservative care is recommended by the most recent studies. Functional rehabilitation protocols should be used regardless of treatment decisions. Although the best protocol is still being debated, it is clear that early weight bearing is paramount to outcome and patient satisfaction.

REFERENCES

1. Huttunen T, Kannus P, Rolf C, et al. Acute Achilles tendon ruptures: incidence of injury and surgery in Sweden between 2001 and 2012. Am J Sports Med 2014; 42(10):2419–23.
2. Lantto I, Heikkinen J, Flinkkila T, et al. Epidemiology of Achilles tendon ruptures: increasing incidence over a 33-year period. Scand J Med Sci Sports 2015;25:133–8.
3. Maffulli N, Waterston SW, Squair J, et al. Changing incidence of Achilles tendon rupture in Scotland: a 15-year study. Clin J Sport Med 1999;9(3):157–60.
4. Nyyssonen T, Luthje P, Kroger H. The increasing incidence and difference in sex distribution of Achilles tendon rupture in Finland in 1987–1999. Scand J Surg 2008;97(3):272–5.
5. Raikin SM, Garras DN, Krapchev PV. Achilles tendon injuries in a United States population. Foot Ankle Int 2013;34(4):475–80.
6. Thevendran G, Sarraf KM, Patel NK, et al. The ruptured Achilles tendon: a current overview from biology of rupture to treatment. Musculoskelet Surg 2013;9:9–20.
7. Cetti R, Christensen S-E, Ejsted R, et al. Operative versus nonoperative treatment of Achilles tendon rupture. A prospective randomized study and review of the literature. Am J Sports Med 1993;21(6):791–9.
8. Khan RJ, Fick D, Keogh A, et al. Treatment of acute Achilles tendon ruptures: a meta-analysis of randomized, controlled trials. J Bone Joint Surg Am 2005; 87(10):2202–10.
9. Lynch RM. Achilles tendon rupture: surgical versus nonsurgical treatment. Accid Emerg Nurs 2004;12:149–58.
10. Moller M, Movin T, Granhed H, et al. Acute rupture of tendon Achillis: a prospective randomised study of comparison between surgical and nonsurgical treatment. J Bone Joint Surg Br 2001;83:843–8.
11. Roberts CP, Palmer S, Vince A, et al. Dynamised cast management of Achilles tendon ruptures. Injury 2001;32:423–6.
12. Saw Y, Baltzopoulos V, Lim A, et al. Early mobilisation after operative repair of ruptured Achilles tendon. Injury 1993;24(7):479–84.

13. Wong J, Barrass V, Maffulli N. Quantitative review of operative and nonoperative management of Achilles tendon ruptures. Am J Sports Med 2002;30:565–75.
14. Keating JF, Will EM. Operative versus non-operative treatment of acute rupture of tendo Achillis: a prospective randomised evaluation of functional outcome. J Bone Joint Surg Br 2011;93(8):1071–8.
15. Nilsson-Helander K, Silbernagel KG, Thomeé R, et al. Acute Achilles tendon rupture: a randomized, controlled study comparing surgical and nonsurgical treatments using validated outcome measures. Am J Sports Med 2010;38(11):2186–93.
16. Soroceanu A, Sidhwa F, Aarabi S, et al. Surgical versus nonsurgical treatment of acute Achilles tendon rupture: a meta-analysis of randomized trials. Am J Sports Med 2012;40(9):2154–60.
17. Twaddle BC, Poon P. Early motion for Achilles tendon ruptures: is surgery important? A randomized, prospective study. Am J Sports Med 2007;35(12):2033–8.
18. Willits K, Amendola A, Bryant D, et al. Operative versus nonoperative treatment of acute Achilles tendon ruptures: a multicenter randomized trial using accelerated functional rehabilitation. J Bone Joint Surg Am 2010;92(17):2767–75.
19. Houshian S, Tscherning T, Riegels-Nielsen P. The epidemiology of Achilles tendon rupture in a Danish county. Injury 1998;29(9):651–4.
20. Jarvinen TAH, Kannus P, Maffulli N, et al. Achilles tendon disorders: etiology and epidemiology. Foot Ankle Clin 2005;10(2):255–66.
21. Leppilahti J, Puranen J, Orava S. Incidence of achilles tendon rupture. Acta Orthop Scand 1996;67(3):277–9.
22. Levi N. The incidence of Achilles tendon rupture in Copenhagen. Injury 1997;28(4):311–3.
23. Suchak AA, Bostick G, Reid D, et al. The incidence of Achilles tendon ruptures in Edmonton, Canada. Foot Ankle Int 2005;26(11):932–6.
24. Movin T, Ryberg A, McBride D, et al. Acute rupture of the Achilles tendon. Foot Ankle Clin N Am 2005;10:331–56.
25. Moller A, Astron M, Westlin N. Increasing incidence of Achilles tendon rupture. Acta Orthop Scand 1996;67:479–81.
26. Nillius SA, Nilsson BE, Westlin NE. The incidence of Achilles tendon rupture. Acta Orthop Scand 1976;47:118–21.
27. Flik KR, Bush-Joseph CA, Bach BR Jr. Complete rupture of large tendons: risk factors, signs, and definitive treatment. Phys Sportsmed 2005;33(8):19–28, 47.
28. Arner O, Lindholm Å, Orell SR. Histological changes in subcutaneous rupture of the Achilles tendon. A study of 74 cases. Acta Chir Scand 1959;116(5–6):484–90.
29. Komi PV, Fukashiro S, Jarvinen M. Biomechanical loading of Achilles tendon during normal locomotion. Clin Sports Med 1992;11(3):521–31.
30. Barfred T. Experimental rupture of the Achilles tendon. Comparison of various types of experimental rupture in rats. Acta Orthop Scand 1971;42:528–43.
31. Inglis AE, Sculco TP. Surgical repair of ruptures of the tendo Achilles. Clin Orthop Relat Res 1981;156:160–9.
32. Ahmed IM, Lagopoulos M, McConnell P, et al. Blood supply of the Achilles tendon. J Orthop Res 1998;16(5):591–6.
33. Bernard-Beaubois K, Hecquet C, Hayem G, et al. In vitro study of cytotoxicity of quinolones on rabbit tenocytes. Cell Biol Toxicol 1998;14:283–92.
34. Maffulli N, Longo UG, Maffulli GD, et al. Marked pathological changes proximal and distal to the site of rupture in acute Achilles tendon ruptures. Knee Surg Sports Traumatol Arthrosc 2011;19(4):680–7.

35. Maffulli N, Ewen SW, Waterston SW, et al. Tenocytes from ruptured and tendino-pathic Achilles tendons produce greater quantities of type III collagen than teno-cytes from normal Achilles tendons. An in vitro model of human tendon healing. Am J Sports Med 2000;28:499–505.
36. Magnusson SP, Qvortrup K, Larsen JO, et al. Collagen fibril size and crimp morphology in ruptured and intact Achilles tendons. Matrix Biol 2002;21:369–77.
37. Tallon C, Maffulli N, Ewen SWB. Ruptured Achilles tendons are significantly more degenerated than tendinopathic tendons. Med Sci Sports Exerc 2001;33(12): 1983–90.
38. Wilson AM, Goodship AE. Exercise-induced hyperthermia as a possible mecha-nism for tendon degeneration. J Biomech 1994;27(7):899–905.
39. Yoon JH, Brooks RL, Zhao JZ, et al. The effects of enrofloxacin on decorin and glycosaminoglycans in avian tendon cell cultures. Arch Toxicol 2004;78(10): 599–608.
40. Balasubramaniam P, Prathap K. The effect of injection of injection of hydrocorti-sone into rabbit calcaneal tendons. J Bone Joint Surg Br 1972;54(4):729–34.
41. Beskin JL, Sanders RA, Hunter SC, et al. Surgical repair of Achilles tendon rup-tures. Am J Sports Med 1987;15(1):1–8.
42. Gill SS, Gelbke MK, Mattson SL, et al. Fluoroscopically guided corticosteroid in-jection for Achilles tendinopathy. J Bone Joint Surg Am 2004;86-A(4):802–6.
43. Corrao G, Zambon A, Bertu L, et al. Evidence of tendinitis provoked by fluoroqui-nolone treatment: a case-control study. Drug Saf 2006;29(10):889–96.
44. Fisher P. Role of steroids in tendon rupture or disintegration known for decades. Arch Intern Med 2004;164:678.
45. Royer RJ, Pierfitte C, Netter P. Features of tendon disorders with fluoroquinolones. Therapie 1994;49:75–6.
46. Van der Linden PD, Sturkenboom MC, Herings RM, et al. Increased risk of Achil-les tendon rupture with quinolone antibacterial use, especially in elderly patients taking oral corticosteroids. Arch Intern Med 2003;163(15):1801–7.
47. Wise BL, Peloquin C, Choi H, et al. Impact of age, sex, obesity, and steroid use on quinolone-associated tendon disorders. Am J Med 2012;125(12):1228.e23–8.
48. Claessen F, Jan de Vos R, Reijman M, et al. Predictors of primary Achilles tendon ruptures. Sports Med 2014;44:1241–59.
49. Strocchi R, De Pasquale V, Guizzardi S, et al. Human Achilles tendon: morpholog-ical and morphometric variations as a function of age. Foot Ankle 1991;12:100–4.
50. Leppilahti J, Orava S. Total Achilles tendon rupture. A review. Sports Med 1998; 25:79–100.
51. Ballas MT, Tytko J, Mannarino F. Commonly missed orthopedic problems. Am Fam Physician 1998;57:267–74.
52. Inglis AE, Scott WN, Sculco TP, et al. Ruptures of the tendo Achillis. An objective assessment of surgical and non-surgical treatment. J Bone Joint Surg Am 1976; 58:990–3.
53. Jozsa L, Kvist M, Balint BJ, et al. The role of recreational sport activity in Achilles tendon rupture. A clinical, pathoanatomical, and sociological study of 292 cases. Am J Sports Med 1989;17:338–43.
54. Christensen B. Rupture of the Achilles tendon. Analysis of 57 cases. Acta Chir Scand 1953;106:50–60.
55. Maffulli N. The clinical diagnosis of subcutaneous tear of the Achilles tendon. Am J Sports Med 1998;26(2):266–70.
56. Simmonds FA. The diagnosis of the ruptured Achilles tendon. Practitioner 1957; 179:56–8.

57. Thompson TC. A test for rupture of the tendo Achillis. Acta Orthop Scand 1962; 32:461–5.
58. Thompson TC, Doherty JC. Spontaneous rupture of Achilles: a new clinical diagnostic test. J Trauma 1962;2:126–9.
59. Scott BW, al Chalabi A. How the Simmonds-Thompson test works. J Bone Joint Surg Br 1992;74:314–5.
60. Matles AL. Rupture of the tendo Achilles. Another diagnostic sign. Bull Hosp Joint Dis 1975;36:48–51.
61. Copeland SA. Rupture of the Achilles tendon: a new clinical test. Ann R Coll Surg Engl 1990;72:270–1.
62. O'Brien T. The needle test for complete rupture of the Achilles tendon. J Bone Joint Surg Am 1984;66A:1099–101.
63. Reiman M, Burgi C, Strube E, et al. The utility of clinical measures for the diagnosis of Achilles tendon injuries: a systematic review with meta-analysis. J Athl Train 2014;49(6):820–9.
64. American Academy of Orthopaedic Surgeons. The diagnosis and treatment of acute Achilles tendon rupture: guideline and evidence report. 2009. Available at: http://www.aaos.org/research/guidelines/ATRguid eli. Accessed May 20, 2016.
65. Garras D, Raikin S, Bhat S, et al. MRI is unnecessary for diagnosing acute Achilles tendon ruptures. Clin Orthop Relat Res 2012;470:2268–73.
66. Toygar O. Subkutane ruptur der Achillesschne (diagnostik und behandlungsergebnisse). Helv Chir Acta 1947;14:209–31.
67. Barbolini G, Monetti G, Montorsi A, et al. Results with high-definition sonography in the evaluation of Achilles tendon conditions. It J Sports Traumatol 1988;10: 225–34.
68. Fornage BD. Achilles tendon: US examination. Radiology 1986;159:759–64.
69. Maffulli N, Dymond NP, Capasso G. Ultrasonographic findings in subcutaneous rupture of Achilles tendon. J Sports Med Phys Fitness 1989;29:365–8.
70. Dong Q, Fessell D. Achilles tendon ultrasound technique. AJR Am J Roentgenol 2009;193(3):W173. Available at: http://www.ajronline.org/doi/pdf/10.2214/AJR. 09.3111.
71. Longo UG, Petrillo S, Maffulli N, et al. Acute Achilles tendon rupture in athletes. Foot Ankle Clin N Am 2013;18(2):319–38.
72. Weber M, Niemann M, Lanz R, et al. Nonoperative treatment of the acute rupture of the Achilles tendon. Am J Sports Med 2003;31(5):685–91.
73. Schweitzer ME, Karasick D. Imaging of disorders of the Achilles tendon. AJR Am J Roentgenol 2000;175:613–26. Available at: http://www.ajronline.org/doi/pdfplus/10.2214/ajr.175.3.1750613.
74. Coombs R. Prospective trial of conservative and surgical treatment of Achilles tendon rupture. J Bone Joint Surg Br 1981;63B:288.
75. Costa ML, MacMillan K, Halliday D, et al. Randomised controlled trials of immediate weight bearing mobilisation for rupture of the tendo Achillis. J Bone Joint Surg Br 2006;88:69–77.
76. Majewski M, Rickert M, Steinbruck K. Achilles tendon rupture. A prospective study assessing various treatment possibilities. Orthopade 2000;29:670–6.
77. Metz R, Verleisdonk EJ, van der Heijden GJ, et al. Acute Achilles tendon rupture: minimally invasive surgery versus nonoperative treatment with immediate full weightbearing—a randomized controlled trial. Am J Sports Med 2008;36: 1688–94.
78. Nistor L. Surgical and non-surgical treatment of Achilles tendon rupture. A prospective randomized study. J Bone Joint Surg Am 1981;63:394–9.

79. Schroeder D, Lehmann M, Steinbrueck K. Treatment of acute Achilles tendon ruptures: open vs. percutaneous repair vs. conservative treatment. A Prospective Randomized Study. Orthop Trans 1997;21:1228.

80. Thermann H, Zwipp H, Tscherne H. Functional treatment concept of acute rupture of the Achilles tendon. 2 years results of a prospective randomized study. Unfallchirurg 1995;98:21–32.

81. Bhandari M, Guyatt G, Siddiqui F, et al. Treatment of acute Achilles tendon ruptures: a systematic overview and metaanalysis. Clin Orthop Relat Res 2002;(400):190–200.

82. Khan RJ, Carey Smith RL. Surgical interventions for treating acute Achilles tendon ruptures. Cochrane Database Syst Rev 2010;(9):CD003674.

83. Wilkins R, Bisson LJ. Operative versus nonoperative management of acute Achilles tendon ruptures: a quantitative systematic review of randomized controlled trials. Am J Sports Med 2012;40:2154–60.

84. Jiang N, Wang B, Chen A, et al. Operative versus nonoperative treatment for acute Achilles tendon rupture: a meta-analysis based on current evidence. Int Orthop 2012;36:765–73.

85. Zhao HM, Yu GR, Yang YF, et al. Outcomes and complications of operative versus non-operative treatment of acute Achilles tendon rupture: a meta-analysis. Chin Med J (Engl) 2011;124:4050–5.

86. van der Eng DM, Schepers T, Goslings JC, et al. Rerupture rate after early weight-bearing in operative versus conservative treatment of Achilles tendon ruptures: a meta-analysis. J Foot Ankle Surg 2013;52:622–8.

87. Aspenberg P. Stimulation of tendon repair: mechanical loading, GDFs and platelets. A mini-review. Int Orthop 2007;31(6):783–9.

88. Gelberman RH, Woo SL-Y. The physiological basis for application of controlled stress in the rehabilitation of flexor tendon injuries. J Hand Ther 1989;2(2):66–70.

89. Lin TW, Cardenas L, Soslowsky LJLJ. Biomechanics of tendon injury and repair. J Biomech 2004;37(6):865–77.

90. Matsumoto F, Trudel G, Uhthoff HK, et al. Mechanical effects of immobilization on the Achilles tendon. Arch Phys Med Rehabil 2003;84(5):662–7.

91. Strickland JW. The scientific basis for advances in flexor tendon surgery. J Hand Ther 2005;18(2):94–110.

92. Eliasson P, Andersson T, Hammerman M, et al. Primary gene response to mechanical loading in healing rat Achilles tendons. J Appl Physiol (1985) 2013; 114(11):1519–26.

93. Zhang H, Tang H, He Q, et al. Surgical versus conservative intervention for acute Achilles tendon rupture: a PRISMA-Compliant systematic review of overlapping meta-analyses. Medicine 2015;94(45):1–7.

94. Cooper MT. Acute Achilles tendon ruptures: does surgery offer superior results (and other confusion issues). Clin Sports Med 2015;34:595–606.

95. Hutchison AM, Topliss C, Beard D, et al. The treatment of a rupture of the Achilles tendon using a dedicated management programme. Bone Joint J 2015;97: 510–5.

96. Ecker TM, Bremer AK, Krause FG, et al. Prospective use of a standardized nonoperative early weightbearing protocol for Achilles tendon rupture, 17 years of experience. Am J Sports Med 2016;44(4):1004–10.

97. Barfod KW, Bencke J, Lauridsen HB, et al. Nonoperative dynamic treatment of acute Achilles tendon rupture: the influence of early weight-bearing on clinical outcome. J Bone Joint Surg Am 2014;96:1497–503.

98. Huang J, Wang C, Ma X, et al. Rehabilitation after surgical treatment of acute Achilles tendon ruptures: a systematic review with meta-analysis. Am J Sports Med 2015;43:1008–16.
99. Brumann M, Baumbach SF, Mutschler W, et al. Accelerated rehabilitation following Achilles tendon repair after acute rupture–development of an evidence based treatment protocol. Injury 2014;45:1782–90.

Acute Rupture Open Repair Techniques

Robert D. Santrock, MD*, Andrew J. Friedmann, MD, Andrew E. Hanselman, MD

KEYWORDS

- Achilles tendon • Acute rupture • Open repair • Limited open • Surgical technique

KEY POINTS

- Achilles tendon ruptures may be treated operatively or nonoperatively; however, the current literature remains controversial.
- Open surgical intervention has historically resulted in lower rerupture rates but higher complication rates.
- Limited open surgical repairs provide adequate end-to-end tendon repair, with improved cosmesis and lower risk for skin complications.

INTRODUCTION

The Achilles tendon is the strongest tendon in the human body and is the main contributor to plantarflexion of the ankle.[1] Consisting of the medial gastrocnemius, lateral gastrocnemius, and soleus, the Achilles tendon is surrounded by a paratenon and attaches to the calcaneal tuberosity. The region, 2 to 6 cm proximal to the calcaneal insertion, has the smallest cross-sectional area and is the most common site of rupture.[2] Approximately 9% of ruptures occur proximally at the musculotendinous junction, 72% occur in the middle portion of the tendon, and 19% occur distally at the tendinous insertion.[3] Ruptures may be partial or complete and are misdiagnosed in 20% to 25% of patients.[4] These injuries are more common in men than in women during the third to fifth decade with an incidence of about 18 per 100,000 persons.[5–7] The injury often involves a noncontact mechanism, such as forceful dorsiflexion of a plantarflexed ankle or vigorous push-off with an extended knee, but may also involve a direct injury, such as laceration or direct blow.[4,6] Most patients experience a sudden snap or shooting pain and are able to be diagnosed by history and physical examination. Imaging studies are not routinely required but may be useful if the diagnosis is questionable. Associated patient factors that may predispose to Achilles rupture

Disclosure: The authors have nothing to disclose.
Department of Orthopaedics, Robert C. Byrd Health Sciences Center, West Virginia University, PO Box 9196 - South, Morgantown, WV 26506, USA
* Corresponding author.
E-mail address: rsantrock@hsc.wvu.edu

include, but are not limited to, fluoroquinolone use, local corticosteroid administration, underlying systemic inflammatory conditions, endocrine dysfunction, and infection.[4]

Historically, operative treatment has been associated with lower rerupture rates and better functional outcomes compared with conservative treatment.[8–10] A Cochrane database meta-analysis in 2010 revealed a rerupture rate of 12.6% with conservative treatment compared with 3.5% with surgical treatment after analyzing 14 different studies.[11] Proponents of surgical intervention also cite the benefits of direct tendon apposition, earlier motion, and earlier weight bearing. However, more recent literature comparing operative and nonoperative intervention is less clear.[12,13] Advocates of nonoperative treatment report lower overall complication rates compared with surgery, excluding rerupture, along with similar patient outcomes if treated with appropriate protocols.[14]

Operative techniques for acute Achilles tendon ruptures can be generalized into 3 categories: open repair, limited open repair, and percutaneous repair. Open Achilles tendon repairs, specifically, have been described by the American Academy of Orthopaedic Surgeons (AAOS) as "a procedure using an extended incision for exposure, allowing visualization of the rupture and tendon to allow direct placement of sutures for repair."[15] Although studies have supported better cosmetic results with limited open or percutaneous repairs, there are concerns for increased rerupture rates and sural nerve injuries compared with open repair.[16] Studies have also shown a remaining tendon gap when using percutaneous techniques that takes longer to disappear on MRI compared with open techniques.[17]

INDICATIONS/CONTRAINDICATIONS

- Indications
  - Acute ruptures (<3 weeks)
  - Young patients
  - Active lifestyle
- Contraindications
  - Chronic ruptures (>3 weeks)
  - Elderly with limited functional demands
  - Tobacco addiction
  - Alcohol addiction
  - Chronic cortisone treatment
  - Vascular disease
  - Severe comorbidities (renal disease)
  - Risk for wound complications
  - Diabetes
  - Neuropathy
  - Local/systemic dermatologic disorders
  - Obesity
  - Sedentary lifestyle

AUTHORS' PREFERRED METHOD FOR ACUTE PRIMARY RUPTURES

The authors work with our referring urgent care centers, emergency departments, and primary care physicians to immediately immobilize acute Achilles tendon ruptures into equinus with a well-padded splint. We recommend that all acute Achilles tendon ruptures be referred to our office within 24 hours if possible.

Acute ruptures with minimal (<2 cm) gap are offered nonoperative treatment or surgical treatment. Surgical treatment is offered only to patients who are nonsmokers and medically appropriate. Those patients who select nonoperative treatment are placed into a functional rehabilitation protocol with expedited weight bearing. For those patients who have a gap greater than 2 cm, and/or prefer surgical treatment, we recommend surgery within 1 week if possible. This system allows minimally invasive techniques to be used. The minimally invasive technique is our preferred surgical treatment. The following description is our preferred surgical sequence:

- Prophylactic intravenous antibiotics and a thigh tourniquet are used
- Position the patient prone with the toes just off the edge of the operating table
- Sterile preparation and draping is performed, followed by the time-out
- The surgeon palpates the defect, and a small (approximately 4 cm) midline incision is made linearly, in line with the Achilles tendon, at the gap
- The incision is carried through the paratenon in the same fashion
- The ruptured ends are identified and grasped with an Alice clamp, and the PARS device (Arthrex, Naples, FL) is inserted within the paratenon, first proximally
- In numerical order, the FiberWire sutures (Arthrex, Naples, FL) are passed percutaneously through the device and tendon
- The sutures are looped by the device, and the device is retracted to the gap, pulling the tails to the gap
- The process is now repeated on the distal side
- The tendon can now be reapproximated by tying the sutures while the foot is in the plantarflexed position
- An epitendinous repair is done with a circumferential, running, locked suture for additional strength
- The paratenon is repaired
- The skin is closed in layers after irrigation
- Sterile bandages and an equinus positioned, well-padded AO (Association of the Study of Internal Fixation) splint is applied

COMPLICATIONS AND MANAGEMENT

Complications in open repair of acute Achilles tendon ruptures can have a severely detrimental effect on the patient's function and mobility. These complications can range from superficial wound infections to deep infections with wound dehiscence to rerupture of the tendon, either partial or total, as well as sural nerve injury.[18–20] The ability to manage complications is important for all foot and ankle surgeons performing open Achilles tendon repairs.

Simple superficial wound infections can be managed with local wound care and oral antibiotics. Deep infections require return to the operating room for irrigation and debridement with or without placement of negative pressure wound therapy. One series by Mosser and colleagues[20] showed improved healing rates with use of negative pressure wound therapy to aid in treatment of deep wound infections in conjunction with intravenous antibiotics and surgical debridement. Deep wound infections often require 6 weeks of intravenous antibiotics appropriate for the isolated organism. Infections and wound complications are increased in patients who are smokers or have other comorbidities that affect blood flow, including diabetes mellitus, renal disease, and peripheral vascular disease. Open repairs of acute Achilles tendon ruptures are normally contraindicated in these patients given the risk of developing these serious complications. A more minimally invasive intervention may be used in these patient populations to potentially avoid this complication.

Rerupture of the repaired Achilles tendon can occur following operative intervention. These injuries can range from partial to complete rerupture of the tendon. MRI is an invaluable tool for diagnosis of partial tears in the Achilles following operative repair. Partial tears of the tendon can easily be managed nonoperatively with cast immobilization and rarely require operative intervention unless the injury propagates to a full rupture of the tendon. Complete rerupture of the tendon usually requires operative intervention. Several techniques can be used to repair the reruptured tendon, including end-to-end anastomosis, V-Y advancement flaps, or fasciotendinous turndowns.

High incidence of deep vein thrombosis (DVT) has been reported in open treatment of Achilles tendon ruptures.[21] One study by Makhdom and colleagues[22] showed the incidence of DVT following Achilles tendon rupture in 115 patients to be 23.4%, with 37% of these being diagnosed before surgical intervention. This finding highlights the importance of thromboprophylaxis following Achilles tendon rupture and subsequent surgery. A high level of suspicion is required when patients present with symptoms. Prevention of DVT should be at the forefront of clinicians' minds when managing acute tendon ruptures.

POSTOPERATIVE MANAGEMENT

Following open repair of the Achilles tendon, the authors immobilize patients for 10 to 14 days in a plantarflexed plaster splint or cast, in order to allow for wound healing. Functional rehabilitation has been shown to provide better outcomes following both operative and nonoperative repair of acute Achilles tendon ruptures.[23] Functional rehabilitation and early range of motion are begun once sutures are removed. The patient is placed in a removable boot with heel wedges, made non–weight bearing, and equinus is advanced 30% each week until the foot is fully plantigrade. At that point, patients are allowed to bear weight fully in the functional brace and functional rehabilitation is continued. The boot remains in place for 6 to 9 weeks postoperatively. The patient is allowed to return to cutting and running sports approximately 6 months postoperatively.

OUTCOMES

Historically, nonoperative management of Achilles tendon rupture was associated with higher rerupture rates, but lower rates of surgical complications.[24] One meta-analysis by Wilkins and Bisson[19] reviewed 8 level 1 studies that showed that a lower rerupture rate was associated with operative treatment, but the surgical complication rate was higher. However, functional rehabilitation and postoperative physical therapy protocols have an impact on return to function and complication rates in patients with acute Achilles tendon ruptures.

One randomized controlled study from 2010 showed rerupture rates to be similar in both the operative and nonoperative groups when functional rehabilitation was performed.[25] One-hundred and forty-two patients were randomized to the operative and nonoperative groups. Results showed similar rerupture rates in both groups and the only difference between the two was that the nonoperative group had slightly lower plantarflexion strength at 2 years from surgery.

Open treatment of acute Achilles ruptures carries with it a high rate of complication and several less invasive techniques have been developed in order to negate these complications. There are several studies in the literature comparing percutaneous repair of the tendon with open procedures. A retrospective cohort study comparing the PARS device with open treatment of acute Achilles ruptures showed a similar complication rate between the two procedures.[18] Although the cosmetic results of limited open and percutaneous techniques have been shown to be superior to open repair, a study by Cretnik and colleagues[16] compared 132 percutaneous repairs with 105 open repairs and found a higher rerupture rate and increased incidence of sural nerve injury.

SUMMARY

Achilles tendon injuries can be serious injuries requiring either operative or nonoperative management. For appropriate surgical candidates, operative intervention may provide lower rerupture rates and adequate end-to-end tendon healing. Our preference is an open Achilles tendon repair, specifically a limited open technique using the PARS device (Arthrex, Naples FL). Postoperatively, we use functional rehabilitation and early range of motion. Although current literature remains controversial regarding operative versus nonoperative management, we have obtained satisfactory results in appropriately chosen surgical candidates.

REFERENCES

1. Sarrafian SK. Anatomy of the foot and ankle. 2nd edition. Philadelphia: Lippincott; 1993.
2. Strocchi R, De Pasquale V, Guizzardi S, et al. Human Achilles tendon: morphological and morphometric variations as a function of age. Foot Ankle 1991;12(2): 100–4.
3. Coughlin MJ. Surgery of the foot and ankle. 7th edition. Mosby; 1999. p. 835–50.
4. Maffulli N. Rupture of the Achilles tendon. J Bone Joint Surg Am 1999;81(7): 1019–31.
5. Leppilahti J, Puranen J, Orava S. Incidence of Achilles tendon rupture. Acta Orthop Scand 1996;67(3):277–9.
6. Longo U, Petrillo S, Maffulli N, et al. Acute Achilles tendon rupture in athletes. Foot Ankle Clin North Am 2013;18:319–38.
7. Nilsson-Helander K, Silbernagel K, Thomee R, et al. Acute Achilles tendon rupture: a randomized, controlled study comparing surgical and nonsurgical treatments using validated outcome measures. Am J Sports Med 2010;38(11): 2186–93.
8. Inglis A, Scott W, Sculco T, et al. Ruptures of the tendo Achillis. J Bone Joint Surg Am 1976;58(7):990–3.
9. Cetti R, Christensen S, Eisted R, et al. Operative versus nonoperative treatment of Achilles tendon rupture: a prospective randomized study and review of the literature. Am J Sports Med 1993;21(6):791–9.
10. Moller M, Movin T, Granhed H, et al. Acute rupture of the tendo Achillis. J Bone Joint Surg Br 2001;83:843–8.
11. Khan R, Carey Smith R. Surgical interventions for treating acute Achilles tendon ruptures (review). Cochrane Database Syst Rev 2010;(9):CD003674.
12. Costa M, MacMillan K, Halliday D, et al. Randomized controlled trials of immediate weight-bearing mobilization for rupture of the tendo Achillis. J Bone Joint Surg Br 2006;88(1):69–77.
13. Weber M, Niemann M, Lanz R, et al. Nonoperative treatment of acute rupture of the Achilles tendon: results of a new protocol and comparison with operative treatment. Am J Sports Med 2003;31(5):685–91.
14. Twaddle B, Poon P. Early motion for Achilles tendon ruptures: is surgery important? Am J Sports Med 2007;35(12):2033–8.
15. Chiodo C, Glazebrook M, Bluman E, et al. Diagnosis and treatment of acute Achilles tendon rupture: AAOS clinical practice guideline summary. J Am Acad Orthop Surg 2010;18:503–10.

16. Cretnik A, Kosanovic M, Smrkolj V. Percutaneous versus open repair of the ruptured Achilles tendon: a comparative study. Am J Sports Med 2005;33(9): 1369–79.
17. Fujikawa A, Kyoto Y, Kawaguchi M, et al. Achilles tendon after percutaneous surgical repair: serial MRI observation of uncomplicated healing. AJR Am J Roentgenol 2007;189:1169–74.
18. Hsu A, Jones C, Cohen B, et al. Clinical outcomes and complications of percutaneous Achilles repair system versus open technique for acute achilles tendon ruptures. Foot Ankle Int 2015;36(11):1279–86.
19. Wilkins R, Bisson L. Operative versus nonoperative management of acute Achilles tendon ruptures: a quantitative systematic review of randomized controlled trials. Am J Sports Med 2012;40(9):2154–60.
20. Mosser P, Kelm J, Konstantino A. Negative pressure wound therapy in the management of late deep infections of Achilles tendon rupture. J Foot Ankle Surg 2015;54:2–6.
21. Lapidus L, Ponzer S, Pettersson H, et al. Symptomatic venous thromboembolism and mortality in orthopaedic surgery – an observational study of 45,968 consecutive cases. BMC Musculoskelet Disord 2013;14:177.
22. Makhdom A, Cota A, Saran N, et al. Incidence of symptomatic deep venous thrombosis after Achilles tendon rupture. J Foot Ankle Surg 2013;52:584–7.
23. Lanto I, Heikkinen J, Flinkkila T, et al. A prospective randomized trial comparing surgical and nonsurgical treatments of acute Achilles tendon ruptures. Am J Sports Med 2016;44(9):2406–14.
24. Erikson B, Mascarenhas R, Bach B, et al. Is operative treatment of Achilles tendon ruptures superior to nonoperative treatment?: A systematic review of overlapping meta-analyses. Orthop J Sports Med 2015;3(4). 2325967115579188.
25. Willits K, Amendola A, Kirkley A, et al. Operative versus nonoperative treatment of acute Achilles tendon ruptures: a multicenter randomized trial using accelerated functional rehabilitation. J Bone Joint Surg Am 2010;92(17):2767–75.

Acute Achilles Rupture Percutaneous Repair
Approach, Materials, Techniques

Jason George DeVries, DPM[a],*, Brandon M. Scharer, DPM[a],
Benjamin J. Summerhays, DPM[b]

KEYWORDS

- PARS • Achillon • Minimally invasive • Trauma • Sports medicine
- Midsubstance speed bridge

KEY POINTS

- Percutaneous repair can offer similar results in regards to rerupture rate as open repair, while minimizing complications.
- Accelerated rehabilitation can and should be instituted safely after percutaneous repair.
- A major concern for percutaneous repair is damage to the sural nerves, and careful planning and instrumentation is paramount to avoid damage to this area.
- Modern techniques for percutaneous Achilles repair and accelerated rehabilitation can offer excellent results in regards to return to activity, better than seen in the past.
- Developing techniques may offer ability for more secure immediate fixation into the calcaneus and allow faster rehabilitation, but more research is needed.

INTRODUCTION

Achilles tendon rupture is a significant injury, and often results from sporting activity in patients younger than 55 years old.[1] Treatment of acute, closed, traumatic ruptures of the Achilles tendon continues to be a controversial topic. Historical nonoperative treatment with extended non–weight bearing in a plantarflexed cast has essentially been abandoned in favor of active rehabilitation.[2,3] A meta-analysis in 2005 found that surgical repair of an acute Achilles tendon rupture leads to a lower rerupture rate compared with nonoperative treatment, and all groups benefitted from accelerated rehabilitation. Open repair was associated with higher complication rates, and this

Financial Disclosure: J.G. DeVries has consulting agreements with Arthrex, Inc and Bioventus.
[a] Orthopedics & Sports Medicine, BayCare Clinic, 2020 Riverside Drive, Green Bay, WI 54301, USA; [b] Orthoaedic Surgery, University of Missouri Health, 1100 Virginia Avenue, Columbia, MO 65212, USA
* Corresponding author.
E-mail address: skisnfeet@hotmail.com

Clin Podiatr Med Surg 34 (2017) 251–262
http://dx.doi.org/10.1016/j.cpm.2016.10.011
podiatric.theclinics.com

was improved with percutaneous methods.[4] Although there has been a recent push toward nonoperative treatment with functional bracing and an accelerated rehabilitation program,[5] there is still recent evidence that operative treatment may lead to a lower rerupture rate.[6,7]

Surgical repair of the ruptured Achilles tendon falls broadly into open or minimally invasive techniques. These two types of repair have been compared in the past. Percutaneous repair of the Achilles tendon has come to represent everything from truly a percutaneous approach, to those with K-wire or endoscopic assistance, to minimally invasive techniques that use specialized instrumentations. These techniques have gone through an evolution over the years. The percutaneous technique was originally described by Ma and Griffith[8] in 1977 as a truly percutaneous repair using a Bunnell-type suture technique through two stab incisions proximally, and then passing the needle through the same holes it exited the skin with distally. Modifications to this technique include various suture patterns, and assistance with K-wires or endoscopy.[9-11] In 2002 the Achillon device (Integra Life Sciences Corporation, Plainsboro, NJ) was reported as a minimally invasive approach through a transverse incision using specialized instrumentation to guide the sutures.[12] This too has gone through an evolution with the addition of channels to guide the suture or techniques to allow for the introduction of locking sutures (percutaneous Achilles repair system [PARS], Arthrex, Inc, Naples, FL).[13,14] Most recently methods have been described and biomechanically studied that tension the proximal portion of the Achilles tendon and secure it in a bridge technique with anchors to the calcaneal tuberosity, spanning the distal stump.[15,16]

The authors present their current recommendations for minimally invasive repair of the acute closed Achilles tendon rupture.

MINIMALLY INVASIVE TECHNIQUES
Preoperative Planning

Approach to the patient begins with a careful clinical examination. Importance is placed on the date of injury. A percutaneous repair should be approached only for acute ruptures. Achilles tendon adhesions with retraction or chronic neglected Achilles tendon ruptures become significantly difficult after 4 weeks. This limits adequate repair with a percutaneous approach.

Clinical examination starts with a supine patient on the examination table to adequately assess neurovascular status and swelling. A standard injury examination should evaluate for concomitant injuries. The patient can then roll to a prone position. Evaluation of both extremities should be performed (**Fig. 1**). Thompson test is used to evaluate Achilles continuity of the involved side. Passive dorsiflexion and plantarflexion should also be used to palpate the level of dell of the Achilles. Careful determination of insertional, mid-substance, or proximal rupture is made. Palpation of the proximal stump is crucial in determining surgical approach. It is more difficult to approach insertional and proximal ruptures of the Achilles with the minimally invasive approach. The authors prefer open surgical approach for these. Mid-substance Achilles surgical approach is discussed in this article.

Adequate soft tissue envelope is crucial to minimize skin complications postoperatively. The procedure is most ideal 7 to 14 days postinjury. To assist in swelling a bulky Jones compression posterior splint is used with the patient non–weight bearing until the operative date.

Operatively, the patient is placed in a well-padded prone position. Both limbs should be draped. Opposite limb draping is used for assessing appropriate Achilles tension during correction.

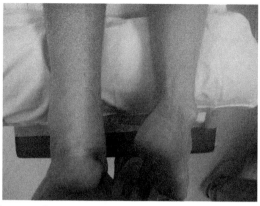

Fig. 1. Clinical evaluation of an acute Achilles tendon rupture. Notice the swelling and lack of definition at the Achilles on the left. Bruising is also noted. Finally, the normal physiologic equinus seen on the right is lost on the left.

Mini-Open Repair with Instrumented Assistance

Over the area of the Achilles rupture the foot is placed in slight dorsiflexion to palpate the delve corresponding to the torn portion of the Achilles. A vertical or transverse incision, 3 cm in length is made. The incision should be made full thickness through the subcutaneous tissue. Care should be taken to not separate the skin and adipose tissue layer. The authors prefer a transverse incision just distal to the proximal stump of the Achilles. Consideration of the longitudinal incision over the transverse incision may allow for abandonment of the minimally invasive techniques if a complication does arise. A scalpel is used to incise through the ruptured paratenon of the Achilles. Heavy irrigation flushes the hematoma. The frayed fibers of the Achilles rupture are identified. A Kocher clamp is used to pull the proximal stump distal through the incision (**Fig. 2**). Manually a finger should be used circumferentially to release proximal adhesions of the stump. One centimeter of the distal portion of the proximal stump may be debrided

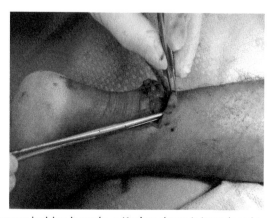

Fig. 2. After transverse incision is made, a Kocher clamp is introduced to grab and pull the Achilles distally. Manual release of any adhesions is performed and the tendon and paratenon are separated. (*Courtesy of* J. Cottom, DPM, Sarasota, FL.)

if the mop ends seem nonviable. This is often not required in the acute setting, and the mop ends interdigitate after repair.

The jig for the system is placed within the paratenon along the proximal portion. Specific care to keep the inner arms of the jig within the paratenon is crucial (**Fig. 3**). Once in place, system-specific suture delivery is performed percutaneously transversely through the proximal stump (**Fig. 4**). The sutures are then pulled through the skin and paratenon and pulled distally (**Fig. 5**). This same technique is then repeated for the distal section. Once both of the ends are each secured with #2 braided nonabsorbable suture, the foot should be placed into 15° to 20° of plantarflexion to bring the ends together and the suture ends are tied. Reinforce this central section with 0 Vicryl suture continuous running from anterior, circumferentially around the tear. Irrigate the wound. Paratenon closure is made if possible with 3–0 monocryl suture. Skin closure is made with 3–0 nylon. A standard dry sterile dressing applied. A well-padded posterior splint with the patient in gravity equinus is used.

Mid-substance Achilles Repair with Calcaneal Anchors

A similar approach to the proximal stump of the tendon is undertaken. Nonabsorbable #2 suture is then used with a suture or jig technique of choice. The proximal stump is now ready. Stab incisions are now made longitudinally with a #15 scalpel to the medial and lateral side of this Achilles insertion on the posterior calcaneus (**Fig. 6**). Specially designed cannulated suture passing instruments from the set are used from distal to proximal. The suture passing device "banana lasso" is passed within the Achilles through the distal stump into the incision (**Fig. 7**). From this level a suture passing wire is passed from distal to proximal in the lasso and the previously placed suture strands of the proximal stump can then be passed to and through the distal stump and out the stab incisions (**Fig. 8**). In the stab incisions a tenodesis or interference anchor is placed in each stab incision of the posterior calcaneus. The foot is then placed in 10° of plantarflexion matching the opposite limb tension. The previous passed suture can then be placed in the anchor and secured (**Fig. 9**). The authors prefer also to oversew 0 Vicryl suture running in a circumferential fashion around the approximated ruptured area. Repeat irrigation is followed by closure of the paratenon with 3–0 monocryl. Subcutaneous closure is made with 3–0 Vicryl. Skin closure is made with 3–0 nylon. A dry sterile dressing applied, followed by a well-padded posterior splint.

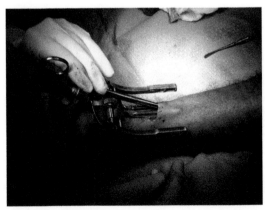

Fig. 3. The Achilles tendon is held firmly with a Kocher clamp and the jig is introduced into the incision and slid within the paratenon alongside the Achilles tendon. (*Courtesy of J. Cottom, DPM, Sarasota, FL.*)

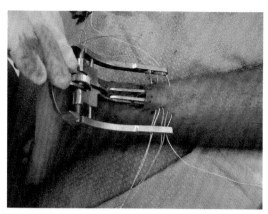

Fig. 4. Using the jig as a guide, sutures are passed percutaneously into the proximal section of the Achilles. Various instrumentation and techniques may or may not allow for locking of the sutures. Slight external rotation decreases the potential for sural nerve injury at this point. (*Courtesy of* J. Cottom, DPM, Sarasota, FL.)

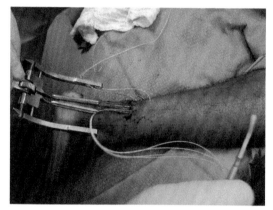

Fig. 5. Once all sutures are passed, the jig is pulled distally. This pulls the sutures through the skin and paratenon and out the incision alongside the Achilles tendon. (*Courtesy of* J. Cottom, DPM, Sarasota, FL.)

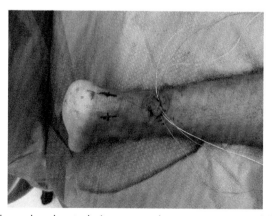

Fig. 6. For the calcaneal anchor technique, once the sutures are passed through the proximal stump, incisions for the anchors are made medially and laterally along the Achilles attachment on the calcaneus. (*Courtesy of* J. Cottom, DPM, Sarasota, FL.)

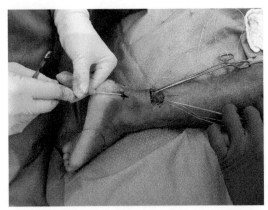

Fig. 7. Through the distal stab incisions, a suture passer is placed into the Achilles tendon at the attachment and passed through the distal stump and out the incision. The lasso is then used to grab the sutures in the proximal stump, and these sutures are then pulled from the proximal stump through the distal stump and out the incisions distally. This is repeated for both sides. (*Courtesy of* J. Cottom, DPM, Sarasota, FL.)

POSTOPERATIVE TREATMENT

Through the developments of percutaneous and minimally invasive incisions the rehabilitation process has changed. Earlier weight bearing and early functional bracing and rehabilitation are key.

The postoperative protocol for our patients includes non–weight bearing in a below-knee plaster splint in the position achieved after surgery. Prophylactic antibiotics and prophylaxis against deep venous thrombosis are given. After 2 weeks, the stitches and splint are removed and the patient is placed in a walker boot with heel wedge. Full weight bearing is encouraged at this time. Full weight bearing without boot protection is allowed at 6 weeks. Functional rehabilitation with physical therapy is started at 2 weeks followed by stationary cycling and swimming at 6 weeks. Eccentric training is added at 12 weeks, and running and sport training allowed at 16 weeks.

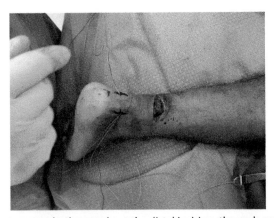

Fig. 8. Once the sutures are both passed out the distal incision, the ends are pulled to ensure that the proximal stump is stable and can be pulled distally. The calcaneus is then prepared with the appropriate-sized drill and tap. (*Courtesy of* J. Cottom, DPM, Sarasota, FL.)

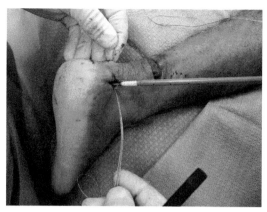

Fig. 9. The foot is placed into approximately 10° of plantarflexion and the sutures are tensioned appropriately. Holding this tension, the sutures are passed into the tenodesis screw and the screw is inserted into the calcaneus. This is repeated for the other side. (*Courtesy of* J. Cottom, DPM, Sarasota, FL.)

Studies have shown that immediate postoperative weight bearing is not detrimental to outcome.[17] Costa and coworkers[18] have shown no evidence of tendon lengthening or increased rerupture rate with immediate weight bearing following surgical repair.

Calder and Saxby[19] in the rehabilitation of repairs using the Achillon (Integra Life Sciences Corporation) jig maintained patients at 20° of plantar flexion for 2 weeks postoperatively and then permitted them to move from neutral to full dorsiflexion for 4 weeks. There were no reruptures in all patients with full return to sporting activities at 6 months.

COMPLICATIONS

Complications are not uncommon. A Cochrane review investigating operative interventions for acute Achilles tendon ruptures reported that operative repair had rerupture rates of 4.4%, wound infection rate of 3.9%, and deep infection rate of 2.2%.[20] The question is whether percutaneous and minimally invasive surgical techniques have a decreased or similar complication rate to open techniques.

The reported complication rates of percutaneous and minimally invasive procedures are inconsistent. There are many variations of technique, which makes it difficult to compare. The original percutaneous method was reported to have a rate of sural nerve injury of up to 13%.[21] Metz and colleagues[22] reported the complications after minimally invasive Achilles repair and found a 36% overall complication rate, with the most frequent complications being sural nerve injury (19%). With sural nerve injury being a common complication of percutaneous and minimally invasive surgery (MIS) Achilles repairs, careful attention to the anatomy and the course of the sural nerve is needed. MacMahon and coworkers[23] evaluated the sural nerve in relation to the Achilles tendon via MRI. They found that externally rotating the proximal end of the rupture while using the MIS devices decreases the risk of sural nerve injury.

OUTCOMES
Percutaneous Approach

A contemporary report of the traditional percutaneous approach was published by Rouvillain and colleagues[24] in 2010, reporting on 60 patients treated in the traditional technique described by Ma and Griffith.[8] The postoperative protocol called for 6 weeks of cast immobilization with progressive weight bearing in the last 3 weeks. There were only two reruptures, one infection, and no sural nerve injuries. Return to work was reported as 85 days, with return to sports at 5 months. Maffuli and colleagues[25] in 2010 reported on the outcomes in 35 patients older than 65 treated in this manner. Of those that ruptured the tendon during sports-related activity, only 50% (12 of 24 patients) returned to this activity. There was an 11% incidence of superficial infection, 11% sural nerve injury, and 7% development of deep vein thrombosis. A recent review of 13 studies encompassing a total of 670 patients evaluated the percutaneous repair in an athletic population. The rerupture rate was 2.1%, and the rate of deep venous thrombosis was 0.6%. Patients were able to return to their previous level of athletic activity in 78% to 84% of the injuries, and back to some level of sporting activity in 91.4%.[26]

Mini-Open Approach

The Achillon mini-open technique has been evaluated in several prospective studies. In 2002 a prospective multicenter study was undertaken and the results of 82 patients were reported. The results in this report were exceptionally good with no wound problems, no infections, and no sural nerve disturbances. All patients returned to previous sporting levels and the mean American Orthopedic Foot and Ankle Society score postoperatively was 96. Three patients were reported to have a rerupture fixed with open repair, and these reruptures were related to either noncompliance or a new injury.[12] Another prospective study in 2005 of 46 patients had an average American Orthopedic Foot and Ankle Society score of 98 at 6 months and an average return to work of 22 days. Only one patient had a superficial infection, and two patients had transient sural nerve irritation.[27] A review of eight studies encompassing 253 patients had an overall complication rate of 8.3%, with a rerupture rate of 3.2% and sural nerve damage in 1.2% of patients.[28]

No clinical outcome measures are currently published on the mini-open technique to tension the proximal Achilles tendon by spanning the distal stump and anchoring to the calcaneus.[15] A biomechanical comparison of an open repair and three mini-open techniques found that all mini-open techniques had more elongation than the open repair when subjected to cyclical loading. The midsubstance SpeedBridge (Arthrex, Inc) technique was found to have no statistically significant difference when subjected to the other minimally invasive techniques in cyclical loading.[16]

Open Versus Percutaneous Approaches

Patient outcomes and complications of open versus minimally invasive Achilles tendon repair have been reported. In a study in 2008 by Gigante and colleagues[29] 40 patients were operatively treated for acute Achilles tendon ruptures, and randomized to receive open repair or percutaneous repair with a proprietary device. Using a variety of clinical and imaging criteria, the authors concluded that the percutaneous repair method was preferred. A retrospective review of 32 patients performed in 2012 compared 15 patients with an open repair with 17 patients with an instrumented percutaneous repair. The authors again recommended percutaneous repair to traditional open repair.[30] Two large retrospective comparative studies also came to the same conclusion. Cretnik and colleagues[31] in 2005 compared 115 patients treated with traditional open repair with 133 patients treated with the classically described percutaneous approach. More recently, Hsu and colleagues[13] in 2015 compared 169 patients with open repair with 101 patients with a modern instrumented technique. Again similar clinical results were reported with fewer complications in the

Table 1
Complication rates of open versus Achillon device

Complications	Open Repair	Achillon
Deep infection	1	0
Superficial infection	3	0
Insertional tendinopathy	0	1
Ankle stiffness	1	0
Hematoma	1	0
Deep venous thrombosis	1	0
Complication percentage (%)	7 (35)	1 (5)

Data from Aktas S, Kocaoglu B. Open versus minimal invasive repair with Achillon device. Foot Ankle Int 2009;30(5):391–7.

percutaneous technique, leading both studies to recommend percutaneous repairs. A meta-analysis of six randomized controlled trials performed in 2011 included six studies, encompassing a total of 277 surgically repaired Achilles tendons (136 with minimally invasive repair and 141 open repair). Their analysis showed similar results in terms or rerupture, adhesions, deep vein thrombosis, and even sural nerve injury. However, the minimally invasive techniques had fewer superficial wound infections, and three times greater patient satisfaction among those that had good to excellent results.[32]

Cretnik and colleagues[31] reported complication rates of 9.7% with percutaneous Achilles repair and 21% for open repair. Aktas and Kocaoglu[33] reported on the complications after minimally invasive Achilles repair (Achillon) at 5% versus 35% for open repair (**Table 1**). Hsu and colleagues[13] reported a 5% complication rate for the PARS (Arthrex, Inc) and 10.6% for open repair (**Table 2**).

RETURN TO FUNCTION

With regards to overall patient outcomes the most important factors are whether the patient can return to baseline physical activities and the time frame to get to that point. Hsu and colleagues[13] reported that 88% of all patients in their study returned to baseline physical activities. The PARS group had 98% return to baseline physical activities at 5 months and 82% at 5 months in the open group. Chiu and colleagues[11] reported

Table 2
Complication rates of open versus PARS device

Complications	Open Repair	PARS
Sural neuritis	5	0
Superficial infection	3	0
Foreign body reaction	0	2
Deep infection	3	0
Superficial wound	7	3
Total complications (%)	18 (10)	5 (5)

Data from Hsu AR, Jones CP, Cohen BE, et al. Clinical outcomes and complications of percutaneous Achilles repair system versus open techniques for acute Achilles tendon ruptures. Foot Ankle Int 2015;36(11):1279–86.

on 19 patients who underwent endoscopy-assisted percutaneous repair of acute Achilles tendon tears; of those patients 95% (18 of 19) returned to their previous level of sporting activity.

Over the last 15 years the reported outcomes have changed significantly with regards to return to sporting activities following an Achilles tendon rupture. Leppilahti and colleagues[34] in 1998 reported only 50% to 60% of elite sportsmen return to pre-injury levels following rupture. This is in part caused by change in surgical techniques and early mobilization and functional rehabilitation.

SUMMARY

Percutaneous and minimally invasive Achilles repair offer good outcomes following Achilles tendon rupture, with less wound complications and hospital stay, and earlier return to activities. There is, however, a risk of iatrogenic sural nerve injury. The authors recommend careful examination intraoperatively of the proximal end of the rupture. With increased awareness and careful appreciation of the anatomy of the sural nerve one can decrease the risk of sural nerve injury.

Early weight bearing and functional rehabilitation is key to the success of Achilles tendon repair. Whether the treatment is open, minimally invasive, or a percutaneous approach, surgeons and recent literature agree that early weight bearing is the key to success.

REFERENCES

1. Raikin SM, Garras DN, Krapchev PV. Achilles tendon injuries in a United States population. Foot Ankle Int 2013;34(4):475–80.
2. Stein SR, Luekens CA. Methods and rationale for closed treatment of Achilles tendon ruptures. Am J Sports Med 1976;4(4):162–9.
3. Keller J, Rasmussen TB. Closed treatment of Achilles tendon rupture. Acta Orthop Scand 1984;55(5):548–50.
4. Khan RJK, Fick D, Keogh A, et al. Treatment of acute Achilles tendon ruptures: a meta-analysis of randomized, controlled trials. J Bone Joint Surg Am 2005; 87-A(10):2202–10.
5. Willits K, Amendola A, Bryant D, et al. Operative versus nonoperative treatment of acute Achilles tendon ruptures: a multicenter randomized trial using accelerated functional rehabilitation. J Bone Joint Surg Am 2010;92-A(17):2767–75.
6. Nilsson-Helander K, Silbernagel KG, Thomee R, et al. Acute Achilles tendon rupture: a randomized, controlled study comparing surgical and nonsurgical treatments using validated outcome measures. Am J Sports Med 2010;38(11): 2186–93.
7. Jiang N, Wang B, Chen A, et al. Operative versus nonoperative treatment for acute Achilles tendon rupture: a meta-analysis based on current evidence. Int Orthop 2012;36(4):765–73.
8. Ma GW, Griffith TG. Percutaneous repair of acute closed ruptured Achilles tendon: a new technique. Clin Orthop Relat Res 1977;128:247–55.
9. Webb JM, Bannister GC. Percutaneous repair of the ruptured tendo Achillis. J Bone Joint Surg Br 1999;81-B:877–80.
10. He ZY, Chai MX, Liu YJ, et al. Percutaneous repair technique for acute Achilles tendon rupture with assistance of Kirschner wire. Orthop Surg 2015;7(4):359–63.
11. Chiu CH, Yeh WL, Tsai MC, et al. Endoscopy-assisted percutaneous repair of acute Achilles tendon tears. Foot Ankle Int 2013;34(8):1168–76.

12. Assal M, Jung M, Stern R, et al. Limited open repair of Achilles tendon ruptures: a technique with a new instrument and findings of a prospective multicenter study. J Bone Joint Surg Am 2002;84-A:161–70.
13. Hsu AR, Jones CP, Cohen BE, et al. Clinical outcomes and complications of percutaneous Achilles repair system versus open techniques for acute Achilles tendon ruptures. Foot Ankle Int 2015;36(11):1279–86.
14. Chen H, Ji X, Zhang Q, et al. Channel-assisted minimally invasive repair of acute Achilles tendon rupture. J Orthop Surg Res 2015;10:167–72.
15. Hegewald KW, Doyle MD, Todd NW, et al. Minimally invasive approach to Achilles tendon pathology. J Foot Ankle Surg 2016;55:166–8.
16. Clanton TO, Haytmanek T, Williams BT, et al. A biomechanical comparison of an open repair and 3 minimally invasive percutaneous Achilles tendon repair techniques during simulated progressive rehabilitation protocol. Am J Sports Med 2015;43(8):1957–64.
17. Maffulli N, Tallon C, Wong J, et al. Early weightbearing and ankle mobilization after open repair of acute mid-substance tears of the Achilles tendon. Am J Sports Med 2003;31:692–700.
18. Costa ML, MacMillan K, Halliday D, et al. Randomised controlled trials of immediate weight bearing mobilization for rupture of the tendon Achillis. J Bone Joint Surg Br 2006;88:69–77.
19. Calder JD, Saxby TS. Early, active rehabilitation following mini-open repair of Achilles tendon ruptures: a prospective study. Injury 2003;34:874–6.
20. Jones MP, Khan RJ, Carey Smith RL. Surgical interventions for treating acute Achilles tendon rupture: key findings from a recent Cochrane review. J Bone Joint Surg Am 2012;94-A(12):e88.
21. Klein W, Lang DM, Saleh M. The use of the Ma-Griffith technique for percutaneous repair of fresh ruptured tendo Achillis. Chir Organi Mov 1991;76:223–8 [in English, Italian].
22. Metz R, Van der Heijden GJ, Verleisdonk EJ, et al. Effect of complications after minimally invasive surgical repair of acute Achilles tendon ruptures: report on 211 cases. Am J Sports Med 2011;39(4):820–4.
23. MacMahon A, Deland JT, Do H, et al. MRI evaluation of Achilles tendon rotation and sural nerve anatomy: implications for percutaneous and limited-open Achilles tendon repair. Foot Ankle Int 2016;37:636–43.
24. Rouvillain JL, Navarre R, Labrada-Blanco O, et al. Percutaneous suture of acute Achilles tendon rupture. A study of 60 cases. Acta Orthop Belg 2010;76:237–42.
25. Maffuli N, Longo UG, Ronga M, et al. Favorable outcome of percutaneous repair of Achilles tendon ruptures in the elderly. Clin Orthop Relat Res 2010;468:1039–46.
26. Ververidis AN, Kalifis KG, Touzopoulos P, et al. Percutaneous repair of the Achilles tendon rupture in athletic population. J Orthop 2016;13:57–61.
27. Calder JD, Saxby TS. Early active rehabilitation following mini-open repair of Achilles tendon rupture: a prospective study. Br J Sports Med 2005;39(11):857–9.
28. Bartel AFP, Elliot AD, Roukis TS. Incidence of complications after Achillon mini-open suture system for repair of acute midsubstance Achilles tendon ruptures: a systematic review. J Foot Ankle Surg 2014;53:744–6.
29. Gigante A, Moschini A, Verdenelli A, et al. Open versus percutaneous repair in the treatment of acute Achilles tendon rupture: a randomized prospective study. Knee Surg Sports Traumatol Arthrosc 2008;16(2):204–9.

30. Henriquez H, Munoz R, Carcuro G, et al. Is percutaneous repair better than open repair in acute Achilles tendon rupture? Clin Orthop Relat Res 2012;470(4): 998–1003.
31. Cretnik A, Kosanovic M, Smrkolj V. Percutaneous versus open repair of the ruptured Achilles tendon: a comparative study. Am J Sports Med 2005;33(9): 1369–79.
32. McMahon SE, Smith TO, Hing CB. A meta-analysis of randomised controlled trials comparing conventional to minimally invasive approaches for repair of an Achilles tendon rupture. Foot Ankle Int 2011;17(4):211–7.
33. Aktas S, Kocaoglu B. Open versus minimal invasive repair with Achillon device. Foot Ankle Int 2009;30(5):391–7.
34. Leppilahti J, Forsman K, Puranen J, et al. Outcome and prognostic factors of Achilles rupture repair using a new scoring method. Clin Orthop Relat Res 1998;(346):152–61.

Repair of Neglected Achilles Rupture

Bradly W. Bussewitz, DPM

KEYWORDS

- Achilles tendon • Neglected Achilles • Repair • FHL

KEY POINTS

- Neglected Achilles tendon ruptures lead to functional deficit and often require surgical repair.
- Advanced surgical techniques beyond end-to-end repair are required to regain power and function.
- Fascial advancements may be combined with local tendon transfer through a single incision.
- Allograft tendon and acellular dermal matrix can be used as augmented or as an isolated repair.
- Patients can expect a functional return to preinjury levels.

INTRODUCTION

The Achilles tendon is made up of a conjoined tendon from the gastrocnemius and the soleus muscle and is the largest tendon in the body. An Achilles tendon rupture typically occurs following an explosive contracture of this triceps surae muscle group. The rupture typically occurs in the watershed area located 5 to 7 cm from the calcaneal insertion site. Less commonly, ruptures occur at the myotendinous junction proximally as well as near the calcaneal osseous junction.

An acutely ruptured Achilles tendon is frequently described as a sensation of getting hit in the area of the Achilles tendon, and often an audible pop is described. Severe pain is usually not present at the time of injury. Inability to push off with vigor on the affected limb may be the most notable acute finding. As a result of these relatively subtle findings, patients may not seek immediate medical care. When patients do seek medical care, the Achilles tendon acute rupture remains one of the most frequently missed injuries in an urgent care or emergency room setting.[1] Patients often lack ongoing pain, and many cannot recall a specific injury. Delayed diagnosis is a primary cause of delayed treatment.

Disclosure Statement: The author has nothing to disclose.
Steindler Orthopedic Clinic, 2751 Northgate Drive, Iowa City, IA 52245-9509, USA
E-mail address: bradly.bussewitz@hotmail.com

Clin Podiatr Med Surg 34 (2017) 263–274
http://dx.doi.org/10.1016/j.cpm.2016.10.012
0891-8422/17/© 2016 Elsevier Inc. All rights reserved.

The neglected Achilles tendon is difficult to define. Some have described ruptures beyond 4 weeks to be neglected.[2] Others have determined a length greater than 6 weeks.[3] Regardless of the length of time that has passed after rupture, if the end-to-end repair is not possible by simply plantarflexing the foot, then the treating surgeon must use additional techniques.

Once diagnosed, acute management, including acute surgical repair or protection and immobilization, leads to an optimized functional return to activities. The goal of treatment is to restore anatomic physiologic tension and strength.[4] If left untreated, the triceps surae continues to contract, leading to potential gapping at the rupture site. The resultant relatively lengthened gap healing allows poor energy translation from the muscle complex to the calcaneus.

The ruptured tendon has been shown to have degenerative histologic changes, including fibrous changes, vascular and cellular alterations, and cell proliferation.[5] The muscle subsequently atrophies and further weakens propulsive strength.[6,7] Ongoing difficulty with push-off strength often first alerts the patient to present for care. Inability to adequately plantarflex, and a reduced stability of the ankle joint occurs if the triceps surae is overlengthened.[8]

Patients typically report a history of difficulty with stairs, unsteady or uneven gait, and a limp during ambulation and during athletics requiring propulsion. Pain at the chronic rupture site is often absent.

Clinical findings of the neglected Achilles rupture include a palpable dell or conversely a palpable bulbous mass at the chronic rupture site. A comparison of the contralateral limb will show increased dorsiflexion and weakness on the rupture side. Similar to an acute rupture, side-by-side comparison while the patient is in the prone position shows the rupture side to be more dorsiflexed at resting tension. In addition, while the patient is prone and the knee flexed to 90°, the rupture side is more dorsiflexed.[9]

It has been shown that operative treatment is superior to conservative care for the symptomatic neglected Achilles tendon rupture.[10] A gap of greater than 2 cm typically exists after debridement, which necessitates a technique beyond direct end-to-end repair. Historically, the size of the gap indicated the repair option.[11,12] A modified version can be found in **Table 1**.

INDICATIONS/CONTRAINDICATIONS

Indications for surgery include symptoms despite failure of conservative efforts, including bracing and physical therapy. Contraindications for surgery include low-functioning individuals, diabetics requiring insulin with peripheral vascular disease, and individuals with extensive soft tissue compromise.

Table 1
Size of defect gap and the recommended repair technique

Tendon Gap	Procedure Recommendation
<2 cm	Direct repair with GSR ± FHL transfer
2–6 cm	V-Y lengthening ± FHL transfer
>6 cm	Turn-down flap ± FHL transfer ± Allograft

PREOPERATIVE PLANNING

The neglected Achilles tendon undergoes changes at the rupture site, requiring extensive debridement and negating end-to-end repair, making repair difficult and requiring advanced techniques. MRI and ultrasound can aid in preoperative planning. The exact location of degenerative tendon and the extent or size of defect can be predicted preoperatively. Suitability of local tendon, such as the flexor hallucis longus (FHL), can also be confirmed for transfer planning.

REPAIR OPTIONS
Flexor Hallucis Longus Transfer (Isolated or Combined)

Local tendon transfer can be used as a stand-alone repair or as an adjunct to fascial advancement or allograft choice (**Figs. 1** and **2**, **Table 2**). Options for local tendon transfer include the FHL, flexor digitorum longus (FDL), and peroneal tendons. Successful use of the peroneal tendon transfer in Achilles tendon ruptures has been documented.[13] However, the peroneal tendon is an important stabilizer of the ankle and is important in eversion power. The FDL has also been reported for use with success.[14]

Due, in part, to a more recently popularized short harvest technique[15] and its location as the most posterior of the medial tendons, the FHL is best suited for replacing the Achilles tendon. In addition, the size of the tendon is typically the largest of the available local tendons, and there is a low morbidity associated with harvesting the FHL. The FHL remains in phase with the Achilles, maintaining its plantarflexory function, and evidence suggests limited loss of first ray function[16] (**Box 1**).

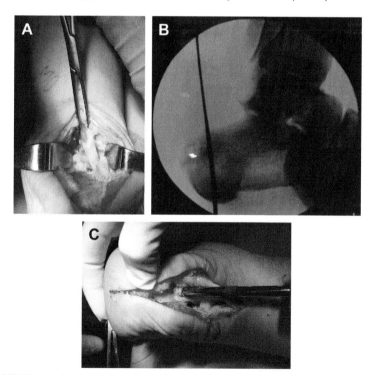

Fig. 1. (*A*) FHL muscle/tendon junction is shown before transecting. (*B*) Intraoperative image showing guidewire placement for transfer. (*C*) FHL tendon passed in bone tunnel in posterior superior calcaneus and anchor inserted.

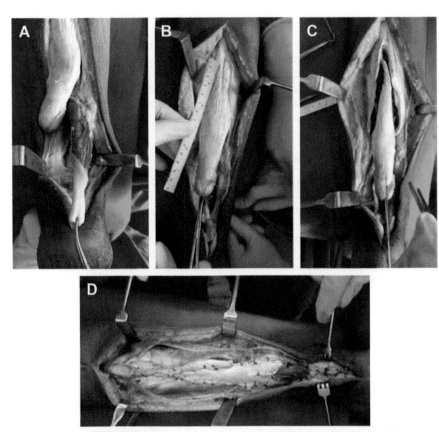

Fig. 2. (*A*) Neglected Achilles stump exposed along with FHL immediately after harvest. (*B*) Marking elongated gastroc-soleol aponeurosis V-Y placement. (*C*) V-Y lengthening actively being tensioned. (*D*) Final V-Y and FHL secured before skin closure. (*Courtesy of* Rahul Tanga, MBBS, Bijapur, India.)

Coull and colleagues[16] showed that, after FHL tendon transfer, there was no pressure change beneath the first metatarsophalangeal joint and no clinically significant functional change evident after harvest. Many reports have shown good or excellent results with short FHL harvest and transfer for Achilles tendinosis and debridement.[16–19]

Table 2 Repair options	
Autologous	Direct repair
Augmentation/allograft	Allograft tendon Acellular dermal graft
Fascial advancement	GSR V-Y lengthening Gastroc-soleol turn-down flap
Local tendon transfer	FHL FDL Peroneal Plantaris

Box 1
Flexor hallucis longus transfer benefits

- Most accessible tendon
- Adequate strength compared with other local tendons
- In-phase posterior group
- Available with single incision via short harvest technique
- Apparent limited loss of first ray strength

Isolated Fascial Advancement (Isolated or Combined)

For tendon gaps up to 6 cm, gastrocnemius recession and V-Y lengthening prove adequate tendon coverage (**Figs. 3** and **4**).[11] Gaps greater than 6 cm typically require turndown gastrocnemius flaps or allograft or synthetic tendon substitutes. Surprisingly, Leitner and colleagues[20] reported a 10-cm gap successfully repaired using an isolated V-Y lengthening.

Us and colleagues[4] described a 22% deficit in peak torque following isolated V-Y lengthening. Kissel and colleagues[21] showed a 30% deficiency, and Elias and colleagues[4,21,22] showed strength is compromised with an isolated V-Y. Adding the FHL to augment the facial advancement may improve postoperative plantarflexory strength.

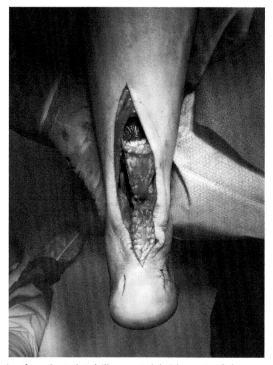

Fig. 3. Direct repair of neglected Achilles post-debridement of degenerative tendon with open GSR.

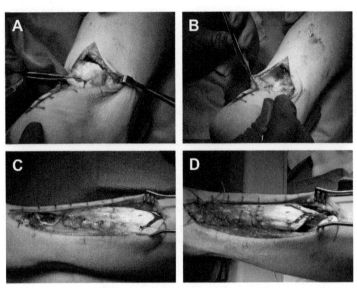

Fig. 4. (A) Degenerative intrasubstance neglected Achilles tendon rupture is visualized. (B) Complete debridement of degenerative tendon. (C) Resulting gap and gastroc-soleol aponeurosis "V" is marked for lengthening. (D) "V" fascial lengthened before "Y" repair.

Multiple turndown flap options have been described for Achilles tendon repairs. The use of local tissue and the extended gap coverage makes the turndown flap appealing for neglected Achilles repair. The flap has also been popularized for augmenting acute repairs.[23–25]

Achilles Allograft and Synthetic Allograft

Recently, Achilles tendon allograft has been reported for extensive gap repair and can include the insertional bony block.[26–28] The entire Achilles can be replaced with this technique and may be valuable when extensive debridement is required (**Fig. 5**).

In addition, an alternative to an Achilles allograft, an acellular human dermal tissue matrix, may be used to bridge the defect or overlaid to support the repair.[29]

A combination of any of the mentioned repair techniques may be used based on surgeon preference and individual repair needs of the patient.

Summary of the Author's Technique

Generally, the author has 2 main strategies. First, if less than 6 cm of length is required, debridement of degenerative tendon and direct repair with proximal lengthening, V-Y if necessary, is the author's preferred technique. He nearly always adds the FHL tendon to aid in optimizing strength to the repair. If greater than 6 cm is required, debridement and turndown flap and/or biologic adjunct combined with FHL tendon transfer are necessary.

Preparation and Patient Positioning

Surgery is typically outpatient with general anesthesia and a popliteal block. Regardless of the chosen repair technique, the patient is placed in standard prone position after anesthesia administration. Preparing and draping both limbs allows intraoperative contralateral limb comparison. A thigh tourniquet is used and allows unrestricted incisional extension to the calf as needed and does not constrict the gastrocnemius muscle. Exsanguinate the limb before tourniquet inflation. The feet should be just at

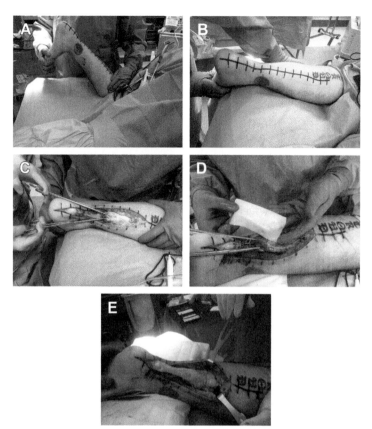

Fig. 5. (*A*) Obvious dell from 6-month-old neglected Achilles rupture when viewing limb from medial side preoperatively. (*B*) Posterior extensile incision planning. Note again the dell is obvious at watershed region. (*C*) Post-debridement gap. (*D*) Tensioning limb with suture and demonstrating acellular graft. (*E*) Final placement of acellular graft and completed repair.

the end of the bed, allowing a bump or stack of towels to aid the surgeon by plantar-flexing the foot as needed during the procedure without assistance and allowing the surgeon to dorsiflex the foot with one's chest with the towels removed.

Surgical Procedure

The following approach addresses Achilles debridement, V-Y lengthening, and FHL transfer. An incision is made midline or slightly medial to midline and may course medial more distally. This facilitates access to the FHL tendon for harvest and best avoids encountering the sural nerve. The paratenon is incised, and the Achilles tendon is accessed. Attempts should be made to make the incision as full thickness as possible to protect the available soft tissue vasculature for this relatively extensile incision.

The degenerative tendon is identified and debrided until more normal-appearing white, glistening collagen is apparent. Again, a preoperative MRI helps guide the surgeon on the expected extent of degenerative appearing tendon. The resulting gap can be measured to determine if enough tendon length remains for a gastroc-soleol release (GSR) or V-Y proximal lengthening, usually less than 6 cm. If the gap is greater than 6 cm, then a turndown flap is used or an allograft may be chosen.

The incision is extended proximally; the gastrocnemius aponeurosis is identified, and a "V" recession is performed. The underlying triceps surae muscle belly will be visualized. Traction is added to the distal end with suture or instrument, exposing the length of the recession, in order to allow end-to-end repair at the debridement site. Krackow suture technique, similar to open acute repair, is performed. Tension should be compared with the contralateral limb. The lengthened aponeurosis is then sutured side to side to complete the "Y."

If the decision is made to perform the FHL short harvest, the incision is deepened on the medial border of the Achilles tendon near the ankle level. Palpation while putting the hallux through range of motion aids in identifying the underlying FHL muscle/tendon and gives a dissection target. The FHL deep fascia is incised longitudinally, and the tendon is followed distally along the medial tuberosity of the calcaneus. The muscle belly to the FHL is the most distal of the posterior muscle group, aiding in the identification process. Again, putting the hallux through sagittal range of motion confirms the FHL tendon before transection.

The underlying calcaneus can serve to protect the tendon during transection. Understanding that the neurovascular bundle is immediately medial and anterior to the FHL at this level helps prevent injury. A blunt retractor can be placed between the neurovascular structures and the FHL for further protection. The hallux and the ankle should be plantarflexed during transection, and the FHL muscle can be pulled proximally to maximize harvest length. Transection of the tendon is typically at the level of the medial malleolus. A number 15 blade or robust curved scissor can safely transect the tendon as distally as possible. Routinely adequate length is obtained with this short harvest technique.

The tendon is pulled proximally from the tarsal canal and a whip-stitch is placed with O-Vicryl at the transected FHL stump in preparation for transfer to the osseous tunnel. The tendon caliper is measured to determine anchor and tunnel size.

The interference screw guidewire with a suture-passing end is inserted from dorsal to plantar in the posterior calcaneus. The start point should be just anterior to the Achilles, and as near the midline as possible, typically slightly medial. The wire is reamed with a matching sized bone tunnel with a cannulated drill after fluoroscopic confirmation of placement. The wire can be passed through plantarly to facilitate ease of tensioning and tendon passing. The anchor, typically 7 to 8 mm in diameter, is placed while keeping traction plantarly on the FHL tendon. Maximum anchor length is preferred to optimize tendon-anchor contact.

Pulling the wire plantarly pulls the suture through the tunnel. The suture is wrapped around a hemostat plantarly, and tension is applied. If the FHL transfer is performed in isolation and the tension is not already established, the foot is plantarflexed comparable to the contralateral limb or approximately 20°.

The posterior superior calcaneus can be resected if impingement is encountered. However, maintenance of the superior cortex may add strength to the repair site by allowing the interference screw to engage cortex in addition to medullary bone.

The foot is taken through range of motion to assess strength and tension. The wound is flushed, and standard closure is performed. A well-padded compressive Jones dressing with posterior splint is placed at completion of the case.

Complication and Management

Complications are rarely reported with repair of the neglected Achilles tendon. Superficial wound infections are the most commonly encountered complication and are managed with a course of oral antibiotics.[30,31]

Postoperative Care

At 2-week follow-up visit, the non-weight-bearing splint and sutures are removed, and a non-weight-bearing cast is applied for 2 weeks. The patient is transitioned to a removable boot at 4 weeks postoperatively with 2 heel wedges, which allow for protected weight-bearing and boot removal for early range-of-motion activities. Wedges are sequentially removed weekly.

Physical therapy is started at 6 weeks after surgery for range of motion and strengthening. Guarding against dorsiflexion beyond neutral is recommended before 8 weeks. The patient is then weaned from a neutral boot per physical therapy and individual patient progression (**Box 2**).

OUTCOMES
Isolated Flexor Hallucis Longus Transfer

Elias and colleagues[32] examined results for FHL transfer and Achilles debridement through a single posterior incision. Thirty-seven of 40 (92.5%) patients at 27-month follow-up could perform 20 single heel raises on the surgical side, and the remaining 3 (7.5%) patients could perform 10. There was no statistically significant difference in independent isokinetic dynamometer plantarflexory strength between the surgical and nonoperative limb. Clinically, no difference was seen in strength. The American Orthopaedic Foot and Ankle Society (AOFAS)–Ankle hindfoot score improved from 56.3/100 to 96.2/100. Thirty-eight of 40 patients rated good or very good results, and 2 of 40 patients rated fair results with no poor ratings. No patients reported weak hallux strength. The original *long* FHL harvest showed a 29.5% plantarflexion weakness when compared with contralateral limb with Cybex testing following FHL transfer.[33]

Flexor Hallucis Longus with V-Y

Combining the fascial advancement and the short FHL harvest has literature-supported success. Elias and colleagues[22] assessed 15 patients at 106-week follow-up. All 15 revealed good or very good satisfaction. A loss of 7.7 (22.3%) N-m plantarflexion torque at 60° per second and a 3.5 (13.5%) N-m loss at 120° per second was reported on the repaired side. They also documented a 5° loss of active range of motion on the repaired side.

V-Y with Turndown Flap

Guclu and colleagues[31] studied 17 patients' long-term results for V-Y lengthening with turndown flap for an average of 7 months after neglected Achilles symptoms. A 6-cm average after-debridement gap was encountered. Following a V-Y with turndown flap, dynamometer testing at 30 and 120° per second revealed a loss of 16% and 17%, respectively. The AOFAS Ankle–hindfoot score improved from 64/100 to 95/100. They reported no reruptures and 1 (11%) superficial postoperative infection.

Box 2
Postoperative course

- 0 to 2 weeks non-weight-bearing posterior splint
- 2 to 4 weeks non-weight-bearing cast
- 4 to 6 weeks protected weight-bearing with heel wedges
  ○ Start physical therapy
- 6 to 12 weeks protected weight-bearing (neutral) and wean from boot at 10 to 12 weeks

Gerdes and colleagues[34] examined strength and functional outcome on average of 4.8 years following turndown Achilles flap augmentation versus direct repair alone. Patients had 41% more tensile strength on the flap side than the simple end-to-end anastomosis.

Gastroc-Soleol Release and Direct Repair Without Augmentation

Porter and colleagues[35] reported 11 patients who had neglected Achilles tendon repair from 4 to 12 weeks after injury with direct repair and GSR. A minimum of 18-month follow-up was recorded. All patients returned to preinjury level of activity. There were no differences in range of motion compared with the contralateral limb. There were no differences when compared with the control group who had acute (less than 4 weeks) repair, and they reported no complications.

Achilles Allograft Repair

Ofili and colleagues[28] recently published Achilles allograft repair for large deficit neglected Achilles repairs. They reported 14 patients with an average 7-cm defect, followed for an average of 16.1 months. Two patients required full bone block grafting. All patients could perform single heel rise at an average of 27 weeks. Patients returned to regular shoe gear at an average of 13.5 weeks. Cienfuegos and colleagues[27] also reported success in a single case of a 10-cm Achilles deficit using an Achilles allograft.

Lee[29] reported no rerupture or recurrent pain in 9 patients with neglected Achilles direct repair, augmented with acellular human dermal allograft.

Several viable repair options are available to the treating surgeon. The addition of the FHL tendon transfer to any of the repair options may mitigate any strength losses accompanying lengthening or allograft options. The ease of a single incision and interference technique makes it a relatively low morbidity addition.

SUMMARY

The neglected Achilles tendon can lead to functional deficits requiring surgical repair. Surgical options typically require advanced repair options beyond end-to-end repair. Popularized single-incision FHL transfer techniques offer stand-alone or augmented repair to the fascial advancement procedures. Allograft options can be used with success as well. Patients can expect an improvement in plantarflexory power and a return to preinjury activities following repair.

REFERENCES

1. Carden DG, Noble J, Chalmers J, et al. Rupture of the calcaneal tendon. The early and late management. J Bone Joint Surg Br 1987;69:416–20.
2. Gabel S, Manoli A. Neglected rupture of the Achilles tendon. Foot Ankle Int 1994; 15:512–7.
3. Pintore E, Barra V, Pintore R, et al. Peroneus brevis tendon transfer in neglected tears of the Achilles tendon. J Trauma 2001;50:71–8.
4. Us AK, Belgin SS, Aydin T, et al. Repair of neglected Achilles tendon rupture: procedures and functional results. Arch Orthop Trauma Surg 1997;116:408–11.
5. Tallon C, Maffulli N, Ewen SW. Ruptured Achilles tendons are significantly more degenerated than tendinopathic tendons. Med Sci Sports Exerc 2001;33: 1983–90.
6. Wapner KL, Hecht PJ, Mills RH. Reconstruction of neglected Achilles tendon injury. Orthop Clin North Am 1995;26:249–63.

7. Abraham E, Pankovich AM. Neglected rupture of the achilles tendon treatment by a V-Y tendinous flap. J Bone Joint Surg Am 1975;57:253–5.
8. Barnes MJ, Hardy AE. Delayed reconstruction of the calcaneal tendon. J Bone Joint Surg Br 1986;68(1):121–4.
9. Matles AL. Rupture of the Achilles. Another diagnostic sign. Bull Hosp Joint Dis 1975;36:48–51.
10. Maffulli N. Management of chronic ruptures of the Achilles tendon. J Bone Joint Surg Am 2008;90:1348–60.
11. Kuwada GT. An update on repair of Achilles tendon rupture. Acute and delayed. J Am Podiatr Med Assoc 1999;89(6):302–6.
12. Myerson MS. Achilles tendon ruptures. Instr Course Lect 1999;48:219–30.
13. Gallant GG, Massie C, Turco VJ. Assessment of eversion and plantar flexion strength after repair of Achilles tendon rupture using peroneus brevis tendon transfer. Am J Orthop 1995;24(3):257–61.
14. Mann RA, Holmes GB, Seale KS, et al. Chronic rupture of the Achilles: a new technique of repair. J Bone Joint Surg Am 1991;73A:214–9.
15. Den Hartog BD. Flexor hallucis longus transfer for chronic Achilles tendinosis. Foot Ankle Int 2003;24:233–7.
16. Coull R, Flavin R, Stephens MM. Flexor hallucis longus transfer: evaluation of postoperative morbidity. Foot Ankle Int 2003;24(12):931–4.
17. Dalton G. Achilles tendon rupture. Foot Ankle Clin N Am 1996;1:225–36.
18. Den Hartog B. Use of proximal flexor hallucis longus transfer in severe calcific Achilles tendinosis. Tech Foot Ankle Surg 2002;1(2):145–50.
19. Wilcox DK, Bohay DR, Anderson JG. Treatment of chronic Achilles tendon disorders with flexor hallucis longus transfer/augmentation. Foot Ankle Int 2000;21(12):1004–10.
20. Leitner A, Voight C, Rahmanzadeh R. Treatment of extensive aseptic defects in old Achilles tendon ruptures: methods and case reports. Foot Ankle 1994;13:176–86.
21. Kissel CG, Blacklidge DK, Crowley DL. Repair of neglected Achilles ruptures: procedure and functional results. J Foot Ankle Surg 1994;33:46–52.
22. Elias I, Besser M, Nazaria LN, et al. Reconstruction for missed or neglected Achilles tendon rupture with V-Y lengthening and flexor hallucis longus tendon transfer through one incision. Foot Ankle Int 2007;28(12):1238–48.
23. Lindholm A. A new method of operation in subcutaneus rupture of the Achilles tendon. Acta Chir Scand 1959;117:261–70.
24. Silfverskiold N. Uber die subkutaneous totale Achillessehnenruptur behander. Acta Chir Scand 1941;84:393–413.
25. Zell RA, Santoro VM. Augmented repair of acute Achilles tendon rupture. Foot Ankle Int 2000;21:469–74.
26. Lepow GM, Green JB. Reconstruction of a neglected Achilles tendon rupture with and Achilles tendon allograft: a case report. J Foot Ankle Surg 2006;45(5):351–5.
27. Cienfuegos A, Holgado MI, Diaz del Rio JM, et al. Chronic Achilles rupture reconstructed with Achilles tendon allograft: a case report. J Foot Ankle Surg 2012;52(1):95–8.
28. Ofili KP, Pollard JD, Schuberth JM. The neglected Achilles tendon rupture repair with allograft: a retrospective review of 14 cases. J Foot Ankle Surg 2016;55:1245–8. Available at: http://www.jfas.org/article/S1067-2516(16)00002-8/fulltext. Accessed June 15, 2016.
29. Lee D. Achilles tendon repair with acellular tissue graft augmentation in neglected ruptures. J Foot Ankle Surg 2007;46:451–5.

30. Maffulli N, Leadbetter WB. Free gracilis tendon graft in neglected tears of the Achilles tendon. Clin J Sport Med 2005;15(2):56–61.
31. Guclu B, Cagdas BH, Yildirim T, et al. Long-term results of chronic Achilles tendon rupture repaired with V-Y tendon plasty and fascia turndown. Foot Ankle Int 2016;37(7):737–42. Available at: http://fai.sagepub.com/content/early/2016/03/31/1071100716642753.full. Accessed June 2016.
32. Elias I, Raikin SM, Besser MP, et al. Outcomes of chronic insertional Achilles tendon using FHL autograft through single incision. Foot Ankle Int 2009;30(3):199–204.
33. Wapner KL, Pavlock GS, Hecht PJ, et al. Repair of chronic Achilles tendon rupture with flexor hallucis longus tendon transfer. Foot Ankle 1993;14:443–9.
34. Gerdes MH, Brown TD, Bell AL, et al. A flap augmentation technique for Achilles tendon repair: postoperative strength and functional outcome. Clin Orthop Relat Res 1992;280:241–6.
35. Porter DA, Mannarino FP, Snead D, et al. Primary repair without augmentation for early neglected Achilles tendon rupture in the recreational athlete. Foot Ankle Int 1997;18(9):557–64.

Surgical Correction of the Achilles Tendon for Diabetic Foot Ulcerations and Charcot Neuroarthropathy

Crystal L. Ramanujam, DPM, MSc, Thomas Zgonis, DPM*

KEYWORDS

- Diabetic Charcot foot • Charcot neuroarthropathy • Achilles tendon
- Diabetic neuropathy • Equinus • Diabetic foot ulcer

KEY POINTS

- Equinus is associated with elevated plantar pressures, which may increase the risk of plantar ulceration in patients with diabetic peripheral neuropathy.
- Diabetic foot ulcerations and Charcot neuroarthropathy have been linked to lower extremity equinus deformity.
- Tendo-Achilles lengthening and gastrocnemius recession are some of the most common surgical procedures addressing the diabetic equinus deformity.

Lower extremity equinus is associated with the development of several diabetic foot pathologic entities. Two of these clinical manifestations, diabetic foot ulceration and Charcot neuroarthropathy (CN), have been linked to tightness or shortening of the Achilles tendon, which can cause equinus contracture, defined as limited ankle joint dorsiflexion specifically less than 10° of passive ankle dorsiflexion with the knee flexed and extended.[1] Equinus is associated with elevated plantar pressures, which may increase the risk of plantar ulceration in patients with diabetic peripheral neuropathy.[2] Additionally, in the presence of peripheral neuropathy, increased plantarflexion of the ankle caused by equinus can affect joint forces and gait patterns leading to diabetic CN changes. In each of these clinical scenarios, surgical lengthening of the Achilles tendon has been used to increase ankle joint dorsiflexion with the notion of

Disclosure: The authors have nothing to disclose. T. Zgonis is the Consulting Editor for the Clinics in Podiatric Medicine and Surgery.
Division of Podiatric Medicine and Surgery, Department of Orthopaedics, University of Texas Health Science Center San Antonio, 7703 Floyd Curl Drive, MSC 7776, San Antonio, TX 78229, USA
* Corresponding author.
E-mail address: zgonis@uthscsa.edu

Clin Podiatr Med Surg 34 (2017) 275–280
http://dx.doi.org/10.1016/j.cpm.2016.10.013
0891-8422/17/© 2016 Elsevier Inc. All rights reserved.

podiatric.theclinics.com

adequately distributing plantar pressures across the foot to prevent recurrent skin and osseous breakdown.

THE ACHILLES TENDON IN PATIENTS WITH DIABETES MELLITUS

Chronic hyperglycemia can cause tissue damage through many pathways.[3] Studies postulate that nonenzymatic glycosylation of collagen in diabetes mellitus can lead to changes within the Achilles tendon resulting in thickening and stiffness. In a rabbit model, Reddy[4] showed that glycation-induced collagen cross-linking was directly associated with increased matrix stiffness of the Achilles tendon. Perhaps the most compelling evidence for the effects of diabetes mellitus on the human Achilles tendon came from a study by Grant and colleagues[5] that compared diabetic and nondiabetic Achilles tendon specimens under electron microscopy. The study found increased packing density of collagen fibrils, decreases in fibrillar diameter, and abnormal fibril morphology in the diabetic Achilles tendons, whereas the nondiabetic Achilles tendons showed normal structural organization. These investigators deduced that such structural changes can contribute to shortening of Achilles tendon-gastrocnemius-soleus-complex, resulting in equinus. Furthermore, on a macroscopic level, a study by Giacomozzi and colleagues[6] found the Achilles tendon in the diabetic patients was statistically thicker than in controls. These investigators concluded this thickening leads to a more rigid foot and ankle that poorly absorbs shock during gait. A study of 1666 consecutive diabetic patients by Lavery and colleagues[7] found that diabetic patients with equinus had higher peak plantar pressures than those without equinus and that those with equinus were associated with a longer duration of diabetes mellitus. Further supporting a link between diabetes mellitus and equinus, a prospective survey of 102 patients by Frykberg and colleagues[8] found a 3-fold risk of equinus in the diabetic population.

Most common conditions in the diabetic foot that are attributed to lower extremity equinus include a forefoot ulceration in the presence of or without partial foot amputation, tendinous or osseous imbalance, and CN. The notion about surgical correction of the equinus deformity in the diabetic patient is based on allowing adequate dorsiflexion at the ankle joint level and, therefore, reducing plantar pressures in the distal aspect of the foot or at the level of CN collapse. Multiple surgical procedures have been proposed to address the equinus deformity in the diabetic patient from a percutaneous tendo-Achilles lengthening (TAL) and gastrocnemius recession to a complete Achilles tenotomy. Special attention must be taken when surgery is performed on the Achilles tendon in the diabetic population, as its complications can cause a serious effect in the overall management of the diabetic foot condition. For instance, overlengthening or rupturing the Achilles tendon after surgical correction of equinus in the diabetic patient may lead into an antalgic gait and development of calcaneal plantar ulcerations that can be quite challenging to heal. In addition, overcorrecting or undercorrecting the equinus deformity during a CN midfoot reconstruction may lead to a surgically induced CN joint, hardware failure, nonunion, malunion, or chronic nonhealing ulcerations.

ACHILLES TENDON SURGERY FOR DIABETIC FOOT ULCERATIONS

Although surgical TAL has become popular in the treatment of diabetic foot ulcerations, there are limited high-level studies in support of this modality. In 2003, Mueller and colleagues[9] published a randomized, controlled trial comparing immobilization in a total-contact cast alone or combined with percutaneous TAL, resulting in healing of all ulcerations in the TAL group and decreased risk of ulcer recurrence compared with immobilization alone. A randomized, controlled trial by Allam[10] in 2006 found similar results but used percutaneous TAL or gastrocnemius recession for their patients; therefore, comparisons between the 2 procedures could not be made.

Laborde[11] performed gastrocnemius recession as the primary treatment of diabetic midfoot ulcerations in 11 patients resulting in no transfer ulcerations. A systematic review by Cychosz and colleagues,[12] looking at gastrocnemius recession for treatment of midfoot and forefoot ulcerations, identified limited evidence in support for this procedure. A systematic review and meta-analysis of Achilles tendon lengthening via TAL or gastrocnemius recession for diabetic foot ulcerations by Dallimore and Kaminski[13] noted complications and adverse events included transfer ulcerations at the heel, wound hematoma, calcaneal gait, and ruptured Achilles tendon; however, the authors of this review concluded that TAL and gastrocnemius recession seem to be effective surgical treatments in healing diabetic foot ulcerations when equinus is present. Interestingly, a prospective study by Salsich and colleagues[14] showed that TAL led to a temporary decrease in active and passive plantar-flexor muscle performance but achieved normal levels of performance by 8 months postoperatively. This finding may indicate the need for close monitoring of possible functional limitations after surgery.

Surgical correction of equinus contracture for forefoot or midfoot diabetic ulcerations can lead to complications such as an overlengthened or ruptured Achilles tendon. This postoperative clinical outcome can have a major impact in the diabetic lower extremity with an antalgic gait or new or recurrent ulcerations and can increase the incidence of surgically induced CN based on altered biomechanical forces in the insensate foot. Percutaneous or open double or triple hemisection TAL or gastrocnemius recession is performed at the appropriate level of the lower extremity, taking care to avoid any associated neurovascular structures. Some of the advantages of performing a TAL include a greater degree of equinus correction, but this may lead to the incidence of overlengthened or ruptured Achilles tendon postoperatively. In contrast, gastrocnemius recession in the diabetic lower extremity has a lesser degree of equinus correction but with a low incidence of rupturing the Achilles tendon during the postoperative period.

When addressing the diabetic neuropathic forefoot or midfoot ulceration, it is highly recommended to first perform the TAL or gastrocnemius recession before the ulcer debridement or resection of the associated underlying osseous deformity. This technique allows the surgeon to adequately achieve the equinus correction first at the desired level and then proceed with the necessary osseous resection underlying the ulcer without facing the implications of over-resecting the osseous deformity, therefore, causing further instability in the diabetic foot. Simultaneous plastic surgery soft tissue closure techniques can also be applied after addressing the underlying osseous deformity and after the initial surgical equinus correction.

ACHILLES TENDON SURGERY FOR THE DIABETIC CHARCOT NEUROARTHROPATHY

Review of the literature finds even fewer high-level studies for surgical lengthening of the Achilles tendon for treatment of diabetic CN of the foot and ankle. A retrospective review by Laborde and colleagues[15] suggested that primary gastrocnemius-soleus recession in patients with midfoot CN could lower rates of persistent, recurrent, and new ulcerations. Early lengthening of the Achilles tendon has also been advocated to minimize development of worsening CN deformity.[16] Surgical lengthening of the Achilles tendon can facilitate reduction or manipulation of the deformity and may allow for better positioning during the surgical reconstruction. Proposed advantages to gastrocnemius recession over TAL in diabetic CN include more controlled soft tissue release, less risk of overlengthening, and less risk of Achilles tendon rupture.

When addressing the diabetic CN foot or ankle deformity, it is highly recommended to first perform the osseous deformity correction by preparing, resecting, manipulating, and temporary fixating the associated joint(s) for arthrodesis before a TAL or gastrocnemius recession (**Fig. 1**). This technique allows the surgeon to adequately estimate the desired equinus correction at the appropriate level before lengthening and being followed by the necessary arthrodesis, stabilization, or exostectomy procedures.

Achilles tenotomy has also been anecdotally reported as an adjunctive procedure in surgical treatment of diabetic foot ulcerations and in diabetic Charcot foot and ankle reconstruction. Currently no high-level studies exist for the use of this procedure in the diabetic foot. Achilles tenotomy is generally reserved for the most severe cases of equinus contracture and has been reported in Charcot ankle or tibiotalocalcaneal

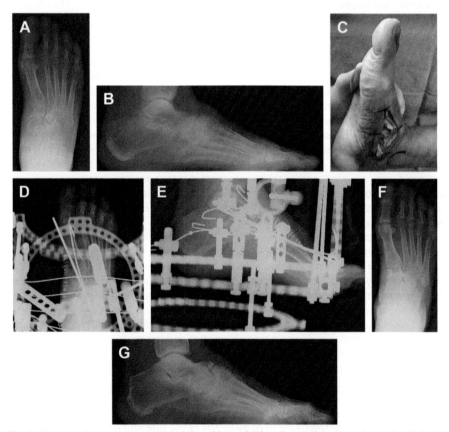

Fig. 1. Preoperative anteroposterior (A) and lateral (B) radiographic views show the diabetic CN deformity at multiple midtarsal joints associated with an equinus contracture. Intraoperative clinical picture (C) shows the resection of the articular joint surfaces and equinus correction with a percutaneous triple hemisection lengthening of the Achilles tendon. This patient underwent an extended medial column arthrodesis with the use of a circular external fixation device (D, E). Postoperative outcome shows the medial column arthrodesis and correction of the equinus deformity at approximately 2-year follow-up (F, G).

arthrodesis.[17] Although the procedure is reported as simple and may achieve significant correction, it has the potential to cause severe complications including calcaneal gait and transfer ulceration.

SURGICAL PROCEDURES

There are several procedures for the treatment of equinus contracture; however, only a few of these are used in most studies regarding diabetic foot ulceration and diabetic CN: (1) TAL, (2) gastrocnemius recession, and (3) Achilles tenotomy.[1,17]

Percutaneous TAL with the use of the Hoke triple hemisection technique is one of the most popular surgical procedures in the treatment of equinus based on its overall simplicity and short operating time.[18] A 2-incision technique has also been used producing similar effects. These lengthening procedures can also be performed through open approaches for more severe contractures; however, they require additional surgical time and may create additional scarring. The main advantage for open lengthening is the ability to have more control over the amount of lengthening accomplished versus the percutaneous approach.

Several procedures have been described for gastrocnemius recession based on anatomic levels, including, but not limited to, those described by Strayer, Vulpius, Baker, and Lamm.[1] Specifically, the Strayer recession involves separation of the gastrocnemius from the soleus just proximal to the gastrocnemius-soleus aponeurosis and allows the transected gastrocnemius tendon to retract proximally.[1] Advantages of the gastrocnemius recession compared with the TAL include a more controlled lengthening, maintenance of plantarflexory strength, and increased vascularity to the surgical site.[17] Finally, an Achilles tenotomy can provide aggressive correction in severe cases of equinus contracture but has a significant risk of calcaneal gait.

Postoperative management with either a posterior lower extremity splint followed by a below-the- knee cast or surgical off-loading with external fixation with strict non–weight bearing status of the affected extremity is crucial in avoiding major complications throughout the patient's recovery. These postoperative off-loading techniques are indicated for either a TAL or gastrocnemius recession for the management of diabetic foot ulcerations or when combined as an adjunct procedure to diabetic CN osseous reconstruction. Immediate non–weight bearing and off-loading of Achilles tendon surgery in the diabetic patient with dense peripheral neuropathy can avoid any postoperative complications, such as rupture and overlengthening.

SUMMARY

The literature clearly shows support for an association between diabetes mellitus and equinus contracture. The pathologic effects of equinus on the diabetic neuropathic foot can contribute to diabetic foot ulcerations and CN; therefore, treatment of this deformity may improve clinical outcomes. Future well-designed research studies on the surgical lengthening of the Achilles tendon in the setting of diabetic foot ulceration or diabetic CN may provide surgeons with better information regarding the efficacy of these procedures.

REFERENCES

1. Chen L, Greisberg J. Achilles lengthening procedures. Foot Ankle Clin 2009;14: 627–37.

2. Zimny S, Schatz H, Pfohl M. The role of limited joint mobility in diabetic patients with an at-risk foot. Diabetes Care 2004;27:942–6.
3. Vlassara H, Brownlee M, Cerami A. Nonenzymatic glycosylation: role in the pathogenesis of diabetic complications. Clin Chem 1986;32S:B37–41.
4. Reddy GK. Cross-linking in collagen by nonenzymatic glycation increases the matrix stiffness in rabbit chilles tendon. Exp Diabesity Res 2004;5:143–53.
5. Grant WP, Sullivan R, Sonenshine DE, et al. Electron microscopic investigation of the effects of diabetes mellitus on the Achilles tendon. J Foot Ankle Surg 1997;36: 272–8.
6. Giacomozzi C, D'Ambrogi E, Uccioli L, et al. Does the thickening of Achilles tendon and plantar fascia contribute to the alteration of diabetic foot loading? Clin Biomech 2005;20:532–9.
7. Lavery LA, Armstrong DG, Boulton AJ, et al. Ankle equinus deformity and its relationship to high plantar pressure in a large population with diabetes mellitus. J Am Podiatr Med Assoc 2002;92:479–82.
8. Frykberg RG, Bowen J, Hall J, et al. Prevalence of equinus in diabetic versus nondiabetic patients. J Am Podiatr Med Assoc 2012;102:84–8.
9. Mueller MJ, Sinacore DR, Hastings MK, et al. Effect of Achilles tendon lengthening on neuropathic plantar ulcers. A randomized clinical trial. J Bone Joint Surg Am 2003;85A:1436–45.
10. Allam AM. Impact of Achilles tendon lengthening (ATL) on the diabetic plantar forefoot ulceration. Egypt J Plast Reconstr Surg 2006;30:43–8.
11. Laborde JM. Midfoot ulcers treated with gastrocnemius-soleus recession. Foot Ankle Int 2009;30:842–6.
12. Cychosz CC, Phisitkul P, Belatti DA, et al. Gastrocnemius recession for foot and ankle conditions in adults: evidence-based recommendations. Foot Ankle Surg 2015;21:77–85.
13. Dallimore SM, Kaminski MR. Tendon lengthening and fascia release for healing and preventing diabetic foot ulcers: a systematic review and meta-analysis. J Foot Ankle Res 2015;8:33.
14. Salsich GB, Mueller MJ, Hastings MK, et al. Effect of Achilles tendon lengthening on ankle muscle performance in people with diabetes mellitus and a neuropathic plantar ulcer. Phys Ther 2005;85:34–43.
15. Laborde JM, Philbin TM, Chandler PJ, et al. Preliminary results of primary gastrocnemius-soleus recession for midfoot charcot arthropathy. Foot Ankle Spec 2016;9:140–4.
16. Hansen ST. Functional reconstruction of the foot and ankle. Philadelphia: Lippincott Williams Wilkins; 2000. p. 246–7.
17. Greenhagen RM, Johnson AR, Bevilacqua NJ. Gastrocnemius recession or tendo-achilles lengthening for equinus deformity in the diabetic foot? Clin Podiatr Med Surg 2012;29:413–24.
18. Hatt RN, Lamphier TA. Triple hemisection: a simplified procedure for lengthening the achilles tendon. N Engl J Med 1947;236:166–9.

Index

Note: Page numbers of article titles are in **boldface** type.

A

Achilles side-to-side repair, 180–181
Achilles tendon pathology
  acute rupture
    conservative treatment of, **229–243**
    epidemiology of, 230–231
    evaluation of, 231–234
    neglected, **263–274**
    open repair for, **245–250**
    percutaneous repair for, **251–262**
    radiography for, 117
    rehabilitation for, 235–238
  anatomic considerations in, 107–109, 115–116
  biomechanics of, 111–112, 144, 209
  diabetic, **275–280**
  differential diagnosis of, 178
  equinus, 207–227, 275–280
  histology of, 109, 130–131
  imaging for. *See* Imaging.
  insertional, **195–205**
  midsubstance
    nonsurgical management of, **137–160**
    percutaneous techniques for, **161–174**
    surgical management of, **175–193**
  noninsertional, **129–136**
  vascular supply in, 109–111
Achilles tenotomy, for diabetic foot, **275–280**
Achillon device, 252, 258
Adherence, to treatment, 151–153
Adventitious bursa, ultrasonography for, 120–121
Allografts, 268, 272
Anatomy, 107–109, 115–116
Ankle plantar flexor muscle performance, 140
Arc sign, 132
Arner sign, 117, 233

B

Banana lasso, 254
Baumann gastrocnemius recession, 211–219
Biomechanics, 144
  of Achilles tendon, 111–112

Clin Podiatr Med Surg 34 (2017) 281–288
http://dx.doi.org/10.1016/S0891-8422(17)30010-1
0891-8422/17

podiatric.theclinics.com

Biomechanics (*continued*)
    of equinus deformity, 209
Blood supply, for Achilles tendon, 109–111
Bony allograft, 268, 272
Bony erosions, radiography for, 117
Bracing, 151
Bump, 176

C

Calcaneal anchors, for rupture repair, 254–255
Calcaneus, bony erosions of, 117
Calcification, 118, 120, 176
Calf-squeeze test, 231–233
Celecoxib, 141, 143
Charcot neuroarthropathy, Achilles tendon surgery, **275–280**
Chung retractor, 214–215
Collagen, in Achilles tendon, 109
Color Doppler, 119
Combination therapies, 149–151
Comorbidities, 138
Complications
    of conservative treatment, 149–151
    of neglected rupture repair, 270
    of open repair, 247–248
    of percutaneous techniques, 164
    of rupture repair, 257, 259
Concentric-eccentric exercise, 144–148
Conservative management
    of acute rupture, **229–243**
    of insertional Achilles tendinopathy, 198–199
    of midsubstance Achilles tendon pathology, **137–160**
        combination, 149–151
        complications of, 149–151
        evaluation in, 138–141
        nonpharmacologic, 144–149
        outcome of, 149–153
        pharmacologic, 141–144
    versus percutaneous techniques, 162, 164
    versus surgery, 178–179
Continuum model, of load-induced tendinopathy, 138
Corticosteroids, 141–143, 150–151, 179, 199
Crepitus, 132

D

Debridement, for neglected rupture repair, 269–270
Deep vein thrombosis, after open repair, 248
Degeneration, of Achilles tendon, 130–132, 178–179
    in insertional tendinopathy, **195–205**
    rupture in, 230

Dermal tissue graft, 268
Diabetic foot ulcerations, surgical correction for, **275–280**
Diclofenac, 141, 143
Direct repair, of neglected rupture, 272
DonJoy AirHeel brace, 151
Dorsiflexion impairment, 140
Dynamometry, isokinetic, 140

E

Eccentric exercise, 144–148, 179
Economics, of imaging, 124–126
Elastography, 122
Enthesopathy, 176
Equinus deformity, **207–227**
    causes of, 207–211
    evaluation of, 209
    in diabetic foot, **275–280**
    lengthening of, 209, 211–212
        complications of, 216
        outcomes of, 218–219
        postoperative care in, 218
        procedure for, 212–218
Exercise, 144–148
Exostosis, retrocalcaneal (insertional Achilles tendinopathy), **195–205**
Extracorporeal shock wave therapy, 150, 163–164, 166–167, 179

F

Fascial advancement, 267–268
Fibular artery, 110
Flexor hallucis longus tendon transfer, 181–183, 186–189, 265–266, 269–271
Flexor hallucis muscle, anatomy of, 116
Foot and Ankle Ability Measure, 152–153
Forefoot, ulceration of, Achilles tendon surgery for, **275–280**

G

Gastrocnemius muscle
    anatomy of, 107–109
    biomechanics of, 111–112
    contracture of, equinus deformity in, **207–227**
    recession of, 187–188, **275–280**
    release of, 272
Genetic factors, 130–131
Glyceryl trinitrate, 143–144, 150
Goniometry, for equinus deformity, 209

H

Haglund deformity (insertional Achilles tendinopathy), **195–205**
Heavy slow resistance exercise, 147–148

Heel lifts, 149
Heel pain, in insertional Achilles tendinopathy, **195–205**
Heel raise test and exercises, 140, 146–147
Hemodynamics, of Achilles tendon, 109–111
Histology, 130–131, 178
History, 138
Hockey stick transducer, 118, 121

I

Imaging, **115–128**, 141. *See also specific disorders and techniques.*
    for acute rupture, 233–234
    for insertional Achilles tendinopathy, 197–198
Infections, after open repair, 247
Injected agents, 141–143, 150–151
    for insertional Achilles tendinopathy, 199
    prolotherapy, 163–164, 167–168
Insertional tendinopathy, **195–205**
Iontophoresis, 149
Ischemia, rupture in, 231
Isokinetic dynamometry, 140

J

Jig, for mini-open repair, 253–254

K

Kager triangle, 116–117, 119
Knee flexion test, 232–233

L

Lactate, 131
Laser therapy, 149
lasma, platelet-rich, 150–151, 163–166
Lengthening procedures
    for diabetic foot, **275–280**
    for equinus deformity, **207–227**
    for neglected rupture, 269–272
Loading exercise, 141–151
Lower Extremity Functional Scale, 152–153
Lyftogt procedure, 168

M

Magnetic resonance imaging, 122–126, 141, 178
    for acute rupture, 234
    for insertional Achilles tendinopathy, 197–198
Manual therapy, 150
Methylprednisolone, 143–144

Metzenbaum scissors, 214
Midfoot, ulceration of, Achilles tendon surgery for, **275–280**
Midsubstance Achilles tendon pathology
    nonsurgical management of, **137–160**
    percutaneous techniques for, **161–174**
    surgical management of, **175–193**
Minimally invasive techniques, for rupture repair, 252–260
Minimum clinically important difference, 152–153
Mini-open repair, with instrumented assistance, 253–254, 258
Mobility, evaluation of, 140

N

Naproxen, 141, 143
Needle test, 232–233
Neovascularization, 119, 131, 178
Neural ingrowth, 131
Neuroarthropathy, Charcot, **275–280**
Night splints, 151
Noninsertional Achilles tendinopathy, **129–136**
Nonsteroidal anti-inflammatory drugs, 141–143, 198–199

O

Open repair, for acute rupture, **245–250,** 252, 258–259
Orthoses, 148–149
Outcomes. *See also specific procedures.*
    of conservative treatment, 151–153
    of percutaneous techniques, **161–174**

P

Pain, 132, 139–140
    in exercise programs, 148
    in insertional Achilles tendinopathy, **195–205**
    in neglected rupture, 263
Palpation, 139–140
Paratenon, anatomy of, 109–110, 116
Paratenon release and excision of intratendinous lesions, 185–186
Paratenonitis
    magnetic resonance imaging for, 123
    ultrasonography for, 120
PARS device, 259
Patient-reported outcome measures, 152–153
Percutaneous techniques, **161–174**
    complications of, 164
    extracorporeal shock wave, 162–164, 166–167, 179
    for rupture repair, 248–249, **251–262**
    vindications for, 162, 164
    modalities for, 162–163
    platelet-rich plasma, 163–166, 179

Percutaneous (*continued*)
    prolotherapy, 163–164, 167–168
    radiofrequency ablation, 163–164, 168–170
    TENEX, 163, 170–171
Pharmacologic treatment, 141–144
Physical therapy, 144–148
    for acute rupture, 235–238
    for insertional Achilles tendinopathy, 198–199
    for neglected rupture repair, 271
Plantar flexor muscle performance, 140
Plantaris muscle
    anatomy of, 107–109
    biomechanics of, 111–112
Platelet-rich plasma, 150–151, 163–166, 179
Plymometric exercise, 146
Polidocanol, 143–144
Posture, evaluation of, 140
Prolotherapy, 163–164, 167–168, 199

R

Radiofrequency ablation, 163–164, 168–170
Radiography, 116–118, 176, 178
    for acute rupture, 233
    for insertional Achilles tendinopathy, 197–198
Reactivity, 138
Rehabilitation, for acute rupture, 235–238, 256–257
Rete ateriosum calcaneare, 110
Retrocalcaneal bursa
    anatomy of, 116
    ultrasonography for, 120–121
Retrocalcaneal bursitis (insertional Achilles tendinopathy), **195–205**
Royal London Hospital test, 133
Rupture
    acute, **229–243, 245–250**
    neglected, **263–274**

S

Sclerosing agents, 141–143, 150–151
Sensitization, 151–153
Shock wave therapy, extracorporeal, 150, 162–164, 166–167, 179
Shoe inserts, 148–149
Side-to-side repair, 180–181
Silfverskiöld maneuver, 209
Soft tissue mobilization, 150
Soleus muscle
    anatomy of, 107–109
    biomechanics of, 111–112
Sonoelastography, 122
SpeedBridge technique, 258

Sphygmomanometer test, 232
Splint
    for acute rupture, 246–249
    for neglected rupture repair, 271
    for rupture repair, 256
    night, 151
Static foot posture, 140
Strayer gastrocnemius recession, 187–188, 211–219
    for diabetic foot, **275–280**
Strength testing, 132
Stretching, 150
Surgical management
    acute rupture, **229–243, 245–250**
    equinus, **207–227**
    insertional tendinopathy, **195–205**
    midsubstance tendinopathy, **175–193**
        complications of, 189
        indications for, 180
        outcomes of, 183–189
        postoperative care for, 189
        procedure for, 180–183
    neglected rupture, **263–274**
Symptoms, 176–177
Synthetic allograft, 268

T

t, rshed region, 116
Taping, 149
Tears
    after open repair, 247–248
    magnetic resonance imaging for, 123
    ultrasonography for, 119–120
Tenderness, 139–140
Tendinitis, definition of, 129
Tendinopathy, definition of, 129–130
Tendon loading exercise, 141–151
TENEX system, 163, 170–171
Thompson test, 252
Tibial artery, posterior, 109–110
Toygar triangle, 117, 233
Training, 144–148
Triamcinolone, 143–144
Triceps surae, anatomy of, 107–109
Trigger points, 150
Turndown flap, for neglected rupture, 271–272

U

Ulcerations, diabetic foot, surgical correction for, **275–280**
Ultrasonic tenotomy (TENEX), 163, 170–171

Ultrasonic therapy, for insertional Achilles tendinopathy, 199
Ultrasonography, 118–126, 141
    for acute rupture, 233–234
    for insertional Achilles tendinopathy, 197–198
    for neglected rupture, 265

V

Vascularization, 109–111
    new (neovascularization), 119, 131, 178
Victorian Institute of Sport Assessment Achilles, 152–153
Video analysis, 140
V-Y lengthening technique, 269–272

W

Wire fixation, for neglected rupture repair, 270

Moving?

Make sure your subscription moves with you!

To notify us of your new address, find your **Clinics Account Number** (located on your mailing label above your name), and contact customer service at:

Email: journalscustomerservice-usa@elsevier.com

800-654-2452 (subscribers in the U.S. & Canada)
314-447-8871 (subscribers outside of the U.S. & Canada)

Fax number: 314-447-8029

Elsevier Health Sciences Division
Subscription Customer Service
3251 Riverport Lane
Maryland Heights, MO 63043

*To ensure uninterrupted delivery of your subscription, please notify us at least 4 weeks in advance of move.

Printed and bound by CPI Group (UK) Ltd, Croydon, CR0 4YY

03/10/2024

01040394-0018